ENDING HOSPITAL READMISSIONS

A Blueprint for SNFs

Barbara Acello, MS, RN

HCPro

Barbara Acello, MS, RN, Author
Adrienne Trivers, Managing Editor
Jamie Carmichael, Associate Group Publisher
Emily Sheahan, Group Publisher
Ken Newman, Cover Designer

Mike Mirabello, Senior Graphic Artist
Matt Sharpe, Production Supervisor
Shane Katz, Art Director
Jean St. Pierre, Senior Director of Operations

Advice given is general. Readers should consult professional counsel for specific legal, ethical, or clinical questions. Arrangements can be made for quantity discounts. For more information, contact:

HCPro, Inc.
75 Sylvan Street, Suite A-101
Danvers, MA 01923
Telephone: 800/650-6787 or 781/639-1872
Fax: 800/639-8511
E-mail: *customerservice@hcpro.com*

Visit HCPro online at: *www.hcpro.com* and *www.hcmarketplace.com*

03/2011
21866

Contents

Introduction ix

Chapter 1: Introduction: Why Are Hospital Readmissions a Problem? 1

Medicare and Senior Healthcare.. 1

Rehospitalization 4

Implications of Rehospitalizations... 7

Rehospitalization and Revenue 8

The Patient Protection and Affordable Care Act 8

Transitional Care... 10

The Bottom Line 12

Why Should I Care? 13

Where to Begin... 14

Chapter 2: Identifying the Origins and Causes of Problematic Transitions.. 17

Interfacility Communication 17

LTCF Concerns 17

Physician Concerns.. 18

Schedule Drug Issues 20

Emergency Department Concerns 21

Patient and Caregiver Concerns... 22

Surprising Information.. 23

Chapter 3: Reasons for Inappropriate Hospitalization and Rehospitalization **25**

Most Common Causes of Inappropriate Rehospitalization 25

Financial Incentives 27

Early Discharge 28

The Weekend Exodus 29

Medical Diagnoses and Conditions That May Predispose Residents to Acute Changes in Condition 35

New Onset Problems Suggesting an Impending Change in Condition 38

Most Common Causes of Inappropriate Rehospitalization 40

Chapter 4: Risk Factors **43**

Identifying Risk Factors 43

The Polypharmacy Problem 47

Medication Reconciliation 50

The Patient Self-Determination Act 52

Why Is This Important? 58

Hospice Care 58

Chapter 5: Medicare Part A Basics **63**

The Medicare Program 63

Observational Hospital Admissions 67

Medicare Paperwork in the Hospital 71

Inpatient Medicare Coverage and the SNF 72

Medicare Level of Care and the LTCF 75

Other Important Reimbursement Issues 81

Trendsetting 86

Documentation 87

Chapter 6: Strategies to Avoid Rehospitalization for Caregivers........ 89

Avoidable Readmissions to the Hospital... 89

Strategies for Reducing Avoidable Readmissions.................................... 89

Standard of Care for Monitoring Residents With Acute Illness or Infection 95

Initial Assessment and Documentation Guidelines for Conditions
for Which Monitoring Is Required.. 99

Specific Responsibilities 101

Change of Condition Communication 104

Chapter 7: Strategies to Avoid Rehospitalization for Managers........107

Managerial Information for Reducing Acute Care Transfers 107

Facility Admissions and Readmissions 107

Commitment.. 108

Establishing or Modifying a Facilitywide Program 109

Philosophy of Care 118

Director of Nursing... 119

Managing Potential Barriers to Success 120

Chapter 8: Essential Elements of Smooth Transitions 125

Transition Initiatives 125

Resident-Centered Transitions... 126

Readiness for Discharge 126

Risk for Readmission or Rehospitalization 128

Communication... 128

Pretransition Issues 129

Risks Associated With Poorly Executed Transitions 133

Teaching.. 136

Preparing Paperwork 138

Advance Directives 138

Medications 139

Other Preparatory Activities... 140

Coordination With Others 141

Home Discharges 142

Other Miscellaneous Issues 142

Steps to Take Immediately Before Discharge 143

Postdischarge Activities.. 143

References..**147**

Chapter 1 Appendix **151**

Facility Definitions.. 153

Twenty Key Conditions 156

Hospital Discharge Planning Requirements 157

Hospitals With the Highest Readmission Rates, 2010 169

Hospitals With the Lowest Readmission Rates, 2010...........................170

Chapter 2 Appendix **171**

Physician Payment Schedules 173

Chapter 3 Appendix **175**

Reportable Laboratory Values...177

Chapter 4 Appendix **183**

Medication Reconciliation Policy and Procedure 185

Medication Discrepancy Tool.. 188

Chapter 5 Appendix **191**

Quality Improvement Organizations 193

Medicare Part A - MDS Assessment Dates.. 195

Medicare Payment Examples 196

Chapter 6 Appendix **197**

Guidelines for Healthcare Provider Notification for Change of Condition 199

Chapter 7 Appendix **227**

Assessment and Documentation Guidelines for
Congestive Heart Failure 229

Assessment and Documentation Guidelines for Myocardial Infarction 232

Survey Audit Checklist.. 235

Transition Coordinator Job Description 248

Chapter 8 Appendix **255**

Discharge Planning and Home Safety... 257

Hand-off Assessment to the Next Level of Care..................................... 267

Admission/Readmission Checklist.. 268

Change of Condition Documentation.. 272

Daily Nurses' Notes 273

Discharge Plan 274

Documentation Checklist: Process Guideline for Acute Change of Condition 275

Fall Prevention Assessment... 278

Intensive Monitoring Log 278

Medication Management Form 279

Nursing Assistant Communication Log... 280

Ending Hospital Readmissions: A Blueprint for SNFs

Nurse/CNA Communication Log 281

QA & A Audit 282

Systems Check for Physician Calls 284

ADL Focused Assessment 285

Warfarin Flow Sheet 288

Tables

Table 1.1 Medicare Beneficiaries With at Least One Covered Event 2

Table 1.2 Medicare Beneficiaries With More Than One Covered Event, 2006 2

Table 1.3 Medicare Spending per LTC Resident, 2006 3

Table 1.4 Breakdown of LTCF Admissions by Facility Type 4

Table 1.5 Average Medicare Spending After LTCF Admission 5

Table 3.1 Average Length of Hospital Stay 29

Table 4.1 Factors Contributing to Rehospitalizations 45

Table 5.1 Most Common Diagnoses in Persons Over 65 66

Table 5.2 Medicare Observation Status 71

Table 5.3 Medicare Part A: MDS Assessment Dates 75

Table 6.1 The M3 Project: Top Ten List 93

Table 6.2 Standard of Care 96

Table 7.1 Brief Comparison of Universal and Standard Precautions 113

Table 8.1 Information to Accompany the Resident on Transfer
to or From Another Facility 130

Table 8.2 HIPAA Myths and Facts 131

Introduction

Reimbursement drives the healthcare system, and you will see how the length of a hospital stay has decreased markedly from 1940 to the present time. The decrease in length of stay corresponds with changes in the Medicare payment system. Originally, Medicare had few limits on the medical costs of hospitalization. However, this eventually proved too expensive, and reimbursement was limited to "reasonable and medically necessary" care. Despite this change, reimbursements were still quite generous and hospital stays were lengthy. In the 1980s, Medicare changed the payment structure from a reimbursement-based model to a prospective payment system with diagnosis-related groups. Prior to this time, physicians were patriarchal and all important. They ran the hospitals, set the rules, and few questioned their decisions to keep patients in the hospital for prolonged periods of time. The balance of power changed markedly with the change in the Medicare payment structure, and hospitals started limiting physician power. One casualty was a marked reduction in the average length of stay. This change in Medicare reimbursement policy affected most of the healthcare providers and insurers in the United States.

As Medicare continued to look for ways to contain costs, they reviewed the expenditures associated with length of stay, admissions, and discharges. One of the most common causes of delayed hospital discharges is due to waiting for a bed in a long-term care facility. This is often due to delays in hospital discharge planning, not inaction by long-term care facilities. Nevertheless, the issue appeared on their radar screen. In the process of studying costs associated with hospital discharges, Medicare also discovered high numbers of preventable readmissions. Thus, they began focusing on ways of reducing costs associated with these two areas.

Ending Hospital Readmissions: A Blueprint for SNFs

It is estimated that Medicare spends $25 billion per year for unnecessary readmissions. At the present time, there are no disincentives for returning residents to the hospital soon after discharge. We can expect to see deterrents in the future because rehospitalization is such a costly issue, and saving Medicare dollars is a priority. Some readmissions are necessary, but many others are not. Caregivers and family members have long expressed concern about the negative effects of hospitalization on elderly persons, such as a deterioration of cognitive status in long-term care elderly. Repeated hospitalizations are stressful as well as physically and emotionally traumatic, and often lead to poor outcomes. There is often no continuity between acute and long-term care facilities, which compounds the difficulty for the residents transitioning between the two. In addition to having adverse effects on the residents, admissions, and discharges are very stressful and time consuming for facility staff. Emergency transfers can be particularly difficult. The numerous small tasks involved in admitting and discharging a resident increase the risk for errors. It stands to reason that preventing unnecessary admissions would be more beneficial and less stressful for residents, their families, and facility staff.

On the surface, the subject of rehospitalization does not seem relevant to long-term care nurses. Have you ever stopped to consider the residents your facility admits, discharges, and readmits? How many of your admissions return to the hospital within a brief period of time? Have you ever analyzed the reasons for the readmissions? Many Charge Nurses and Directors of Nursing accept rehospitalizations as a fact of life. But are they? Some believe that improved monitoring will solve the problem. Is this the only factor? Would an analysis of the readmissions in your facility lead to improvements in care delivery? Since this is an area of governmental focus, it would be wise for facilities to analyze their information and implement corrective action as needed. This book will help long-term care facility staff:

- Understand the financial and quality of care implications associated with rehospitalizations

- Explain why maintaining the census is a priority in long-term care facilities

- Identify priorities and develop protocols and practices for reducing a resident's risk of returning to the hospital after admission to the long-term care facility

- Teach staff the skills needed to help prevent rehospitalization

- Understand the importance of communication and documentation, the role of care plans and clinical care pathways, and the importance of advanced care planning

- Develop effective discharge protocols

- Understand the importance of medication reconciliation and management

- Understand the importance of careful, frequent monitoring of residents who were recently admitted

- Develop protocols for monitoring residents

- Recognize early changes in resident status

- Understand how to ensure residents derive maximum benefit from the Medicare program

- Identify communication problems and enhance communication with other healthcare providers about a resident's change of status

- Identify strategies for preventing rehospitalizations

- Describe methods for ensuring smooth transitions

- Provide effective, individualized postdischarge care

Preventing unnecessary readmissions involves using the nursing process and the information in your book to analyze your facility admissions and discharges and develop a plan to reduce unnecessary readmissions:

- **Assessment phase** – Analyze your admissions, discharges, and reasons for them. Ask yourself these questions: If a resident returns to the hospital, how long did he or she stay in the facility? What is the reason for the rehospitalization? Could it have been avoided? What is the process for discharging the resident to home or a lower level of care? What predischarge planning and teaching are done? How does the facility follow the resident after discharge? Why is postdischarge monitoring important?

- **Planning phase** – After collecting and analyzing data, develop a preliminary plan to reduce unnecessary hospitalizations. Determine what resources are needed. Identify educational needs of staff. Determine whether practices, processes, policies, and procedures need to change. Involve staff at all levels in developing the plan. They are much more likely to make it work if they have an investment in the process.

- **Implementation phase** – Implement the plan. Keep objective records during the implementation phase. The records will be useful when you begin to evaluate the effectiveness of the plan. Do not be disappointed if the plan is not 100% effective. This is normal. Identifying and working through problems encourages growth. Set a target date for evaluating the plan.

- **Evaluation phase** – The frequency of admissions and discharges in your facility will help you determine the target date for evaluating the plan. Facilities with many admissions and discharges will be able to evaluate the plan more quickly than facilities with little resident turnover. When you have collected the necessary information, call a meeting of the original planning committee. Evaluate the effectiveness of the plan based on the information you have collected and comments from the residents, families, and staff. Make modifications as needed and begin again until you have fine tuned your facility processes and the plan is as effective as it can be.

This writer commends and respects those who dedicate their careers to improving quality of life and quality of care for our long-term care facility elderly. Your facility can make a difference in reducing unnecessary rehospitalizations while improving quality of care and the quality of residents' lives. Best wishes on your journey!

Barbara Acello

January 2011

bacello@spamcop.net

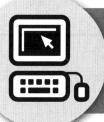

DOWNLOAD YOUR MATERIALS NOW

An informed and proactive nursing home staff is a vital weapon in the struggle to keep residents from being readmitted to the hospital. To assist your facility in reducing rehospitalizations and improve transitions of care, download the tools, forms, and additional materials found in the Appendix of this book. For a complete listing of available tools and forms, reference the Appendix section of the Table of Contents of this book.

www.hcpro.com/downloads/9281

Thank you for purchasing this product!

HCPro

CHAPTER 1

Introduction: Why Are Hospital Readmissions a Problem?

Medicare and Senior Healthcare

The Medicare program pays for the healthcare for most senior citizens in the United States. Fifty-one percent of covered individuals experience at least one Medicare-covered event each year (Table 1.1). Approximately 2.2 million Medicare beneficiaries lived in long-term care facilities sometime during 2006. This is about 6% of the total Medicare population. Residents living in the various types of long-term care facilities account for a disproportionately large portion of the total Medicare spending (17%), with high rates of hospital care, skilled nursing facility (SNF) care, and other Medicare-covered services (Table 1.2). The cost that the Medicare program paid for these services was $25 billion, or 9% of total Medicare spending in 2006 (Table 1.3). This is about twice as much money as Medicare spent for the care of persons not living in facilities.

As much as 40% of the 2006 costs were paid to hospitals for emergency department visits, inpatient and observational admissions, and skilled nursing care. In addition to being costly, hospitalizations often cause untoward physical and mental effects, such as weakness, delirium, and declines in cognitive status. Approximately 600,000 Medicare beneficiaries are admitted to long-term care facilities annually. The average Medicare spending for residents who lived for at least six months after admission in 2003–2006 was more than twice the average monthly spending for those who had lived in the

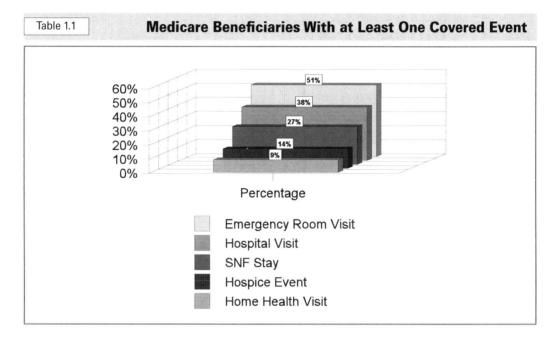

Table 1.1

Medicare Beneficiaries With at Least One Covered Event

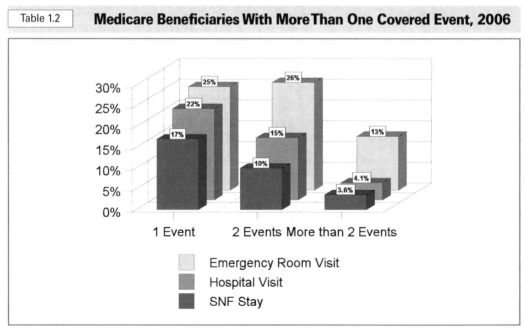

Table 1.2

Medicare Beneficiaries With More Than One Covered Event, 2006

Table 1.3	**Medicare Spending per LTC Resident, 2006**

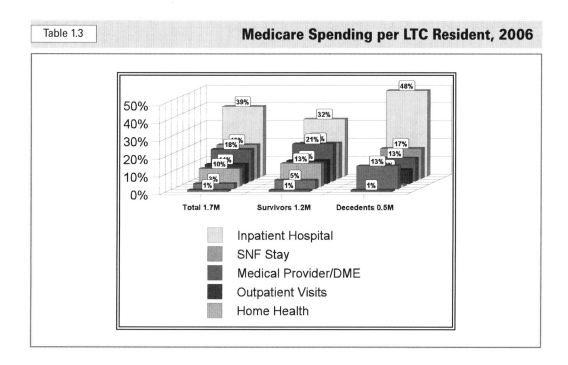

Inpatient Hospital
SNF Stay
Medical Provider/DME
Outpatient Visits
Home Health

facility for a year or more (Table 1.4). Refer to the facility definitions in the Appendix of your book, then review Table 1.4 for a breakdown of admissions by type of facility. As you can see, Medicare spending is much higher immediately after facility admission. One reason for this is readmissions to the hospital.

Recent studies suggest that the incidence of complications can be reduced and many rehospitalizations can be prevented with careful monitoring and attentive care management, medical support in the facility, and better transitions to and from the hospital. Many preventable hospital admissions and readmissions are the result of poor communication.

Table 1.4	Breakdown of LTCF Admissions by Facility Type

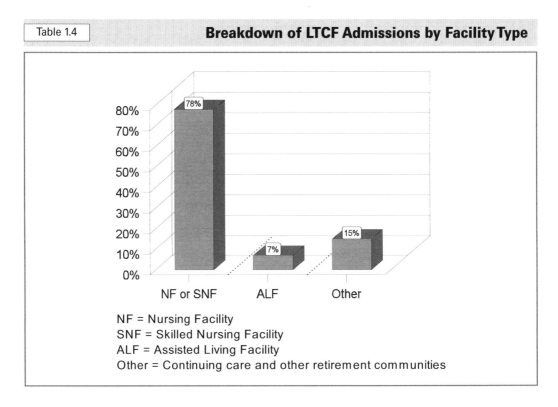

NF = Nursing Facility
SNF = Skilled Nursing Facility
ALF = Assisted Living Facility
Other = Continuing care and other retirement communities

Rehospitalization

The need for containing and reducing healthcare costs has been in the news for quite some time. You have undoubtedly heard that Social Security is running out of money. A significant cause of this problem is hospital readmissions. This refers to patients who are discharged from an acute care hospital and are hospitalized again within 30 days of discharge.

Definitions, facts, and figures

Rehospitalizations are unanticipated, unscheduled readmissions to the hospital that are clinically related to the initial admission. Although the person is typically returned to the original admitting hospital, a rehospitalization occurs when the person is admitted

| Table 1.5 | **Average Medicare Spending After LTCF Admission** |

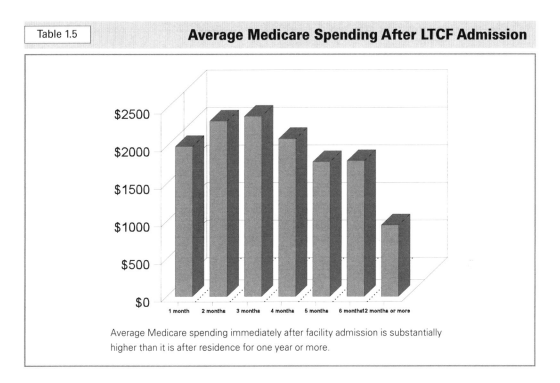

Average Medicare spending immediately after facility admission is substantially higher than it is after residence for one year or more.

to any hospital for treatment of the original condition. This phenomenon is sometimes called bounce back. A newer term is complicated (or complex) transition. Patients who are repeatedly admitted are often called frequent flyers. Very few people want to return to the hospital. Likewise, hospitals do not want their discharged patients to return. It is usually a lose–lose situation for both parties. The facts are abysmal:

- According to the Institute for Healthcare Improvement (IHI), there are about 5 million hospital readmissions annually.

  – Approximately a third of these occur within 90 days of discharge

  – About 46% of these could be prevented

- Estimates vary by year, but 15% to 25% of all Medicare hospitalizations are rehospitalizations.

Ending Hospital Readmissions: A Blueprint for SNFs

- Rehospitalizations account for $15 billion in annual Medicare spending.

- Thirty-four percent of the Medicare beneficiaries were rehospitalized within 90 days.

- 68.9% of patients readmitted or had died within a year.

- Of those admitted to long-term care facilities, 22% to 29% were readmitted to the hospital.

- In 2006, the cost to Medicare associated with SNF rehospitalizations was $4.3 billion, with an average rehospitalization Medicare payment totaling $10,352.

- The death rate for stroke survivors was 26.7% in the first year after hospital discharge. The readmission rate was 56.2%. The overall risk of death or readmission was 61.9%.

- Medicare is collecting readmission data and will calculate a three-year average of readmission rates.

- Hospitals with high rates of rehospitalizations will be financially penalized in the near future.

- The state of Idaho has the lowest incidence of rehospitalizations.

- Rural hospitals have almost twice as many preventable readmissions than urban hospitals.

- About 60% of persons over age 65 had potentially preventable hospital stays.

- Approximately 5.4% of all individuals with private insurance or Medicare coverage were admitted for potentially preventable conditions.

- Men are more likely to be hospitalized for a *chronic* preventable condition than women.

- Men are less likely than women to be hospitalized for a potentially preventable *acute* condition.

- Of all patients, 20% to 40% are rehospitalized at a different hospital.

 - Twenty conditions account for 58% of all episodes of care.

  - Fracture and dislocation of lower extremities and bacterial lung infections are the only two that are acute.

  - The remaining 18 are chronic conditions (i.e., diabetes, chronic obstructive pulmonary disease, congestive heart failure, renal failure). Refer to the list in the Appendix of your book.

  - Ten of these conditions represent the fastest growing costs of care and represented 29% of Medicare spending in 2005.

Implications of Rehospitalizations

In addition to the financial implications facing hospitals, a high incidence of readmissions has the potential for sending a negative message about hospital quality and safety. The Centers for Medicare & Medicaid Services (CMS) Hospital Compare website lists readmission information as one of the indicators of hospital performance. Enlightened consumers may view a high incidence of readmissions as an indicator of unfavorable conditions or care, even if this is not the case. A high rate of rehospitalizations may also suggest:

- Inadequate care for persons with chronic illness

- Failure to plan and deliver the medical services necessary to prevent readmission

- Failure to plan and deliver discharge planning services needed for successful community reentry upon hospital discharge

Ending Hospital Readmissions: A Blueprint for SNFs

Rehospitalization and Revenue

Medicare pays for rehospitalizations, except those in which the person is rehospitalized within 24 hours after discharge for the same condition for which they were originally hospitalized. Even a small reduction in readmissions would save a lot of money for Medicare. Recent policy proposals create payment incentives to reduce the rates of rehospitalization.

Another issue is that readmission rates vary by hospital and geographic region. This suggests that some hospitals and geographic areas do a better job than others at containing readmission rates. Some policymakers believe that reducing readmissions would result in improved quality of care in addition to reducing costs.

The Patient Protection and Affordable Care Act

Medicare has always promoted hospital discharge planning, but has never been particularly successful at containing costs due to improved transitions. No additional funding is provided for comprehensive discharge planning. Medicare has never provided financial incentives or any type of formal structure in the payment system to advance these goals. There has been a great deal of lip service about effective discharge planning, but there were no systematic measures to ensure the discharge plan was effective or that it improved quality. Because of this, discharge planning often does not begin until a utilization review plan has identified a patient for discharge. This is usually late in the admission. If this is the case, the time frame prior to discharge is simply too tight to ensure effective discharge planning and teaching.

Long-term care facilities are required to begin discharge planning at the time of admission. Although the hospital regulation is comparable, discharge planning is often a low priority. Beginning discharge planning on admission is a key step in ensuring all bases are covered. Hospital discharge planning requirements can be found in the Appendix of your book.

In March 2010, President Obama signed into law the Patient Protection and Affordable Care Act (PPACA), as amended by the Healthcare and Education Reconciliation Act. This comprehensive healthcare reform legislation contains provisions that change the Medicare program, including some that are designed to decrease the number of unnecessary hospital readmissions by reducing payment to hospitals with high rates of preventable readmissions. Other portions of this bill are demonstrations and experimental pilots that test reforms to the Medicare payment system for hospitals and other healthcare providers.

The change in the law is planned for implementation in October 2012. Aside from not paying for readmissions within 24 hours of discharge, Medicare will not penalize hospitals further. The October 2012 changes direct Medicare to recover payments for "unnecessary readmissions" within 30 days of discharge if the patient has one of three conditions:

- Heart attack

- Pneumonia

- Heart failure

During the first year of implementation, a hospital's total Medicare payments can be reduced by up to 1%. The total payment reduction is up to 2% the next year and 3% the third year. CMS also plans to add more diseases to the list.

In the future, physicians will also be expected to provide better care, thus keeping patients out of the hospital. Cynics note that developing an incentive program to keep people out of the hospital could cause physicians and hospitals to discharge patients too early because they know they will be paid less. There are also concerns that hospitals will refuse to readmit patients with legitimate medical needs.

After the law changes, CMS plans to penalize "all readmissions" for any reason except planned readmissions, such as those needing additional procedures. Medicare will pay for these scheduled procedures. Although this change will be phased in gradually, the implications of this change in payment are frightening. For example, if a person who was hospitalized for treatment of pneumonia falls and breaks a hip three weeks after discharge, the hospital will be penalized. Although this may seem unfair, Medicare defends this action by noting that counting only rehospitalizations for the same condition would tempt the hospital to modify or alter the condition codes used for billing to avoid a penalty. Medicare hopes to reduce readmissions by at least 25%, which they consider a conservative figure because they believe 30% to 67% of all rehospitalizations can be avoided. A 25% reduction in readmissions would save Medicare over $2 billion in 2011. This figure does not include savings from avoidable emergency room visits and long-term care facility stays.

Transitional Care

Transitional care is coordinated care that ensures continuity. In the hospital it begins immediately after an illness or surgery in anticipation of the person's return home or to a lesser care setting. It is based on a well-developed, interdisciplinary plan of care and the availability of qualified healthcare professionals who are familiar with the patient's clinical status, treatment goals, and preferences. Transitional care also includes patient and family education and coordination of the health professionals involved in the transition. It should include comprehensive discharge planning and posthospital home visits.

Transition of care

Transition of care is the movement of patients between various settings in which care is delivered, different healthcare providers, or different levels of care within the same facility as a person's condition and needs change. Each transition increases the risk of poor care coordination and inadequate communication across settings. The safest transitions are resident-centered. Some provisions of the PPACA will test various changes in care given to persons with chronic illnesses during the original hospitalization, in preparation for and at the time of discharge, and follow-up after discharge as these individuals transition out of the hospital, returning to their homes and long-term care settings.

Transition extends the responsibility of the discharging unit or facility into the new location or level of care. Responsibility of the original care team continues until all questions about the patient are answered and the new caregivers acknowledge the assumption of care. Some progressive hospitals have transitional nurses and transitional coaches who prepare the patient and receiving facility for the transfer, then follow up to address any issues that arise. In any care transition, all professionals who send and receive information must:

- Validate the transfer

- Accept the information

- Clarify discrepancies

- Accurately act on the information in a timely manner

Relocation stress syndrome

Transitioning from one setting to another has the potential for causing or increasing confusion and traumatizing an elderly resident. Signs and symptoms include:

- Increased dependence

- Delirium

- Depression

- Anger

- Withdrawal

- Changes in behavior

Ending Hospital Readmissions: A Blueprint for SNFs

- Changes in sleeping habits

- Feelings of insecurity, loss of trust

- Weight loss (or, less commonly, gain)

- Falls

This is the phenomena known as relocation stress syndrome. Older terms that may still be used are transfer trauma and relocation shock. Relocation stress syndrome is a consequence of the stress and emotional shock caused by an abrupt relocation of a resident from one location or facility to another. Unless a proposed transfer is emergent, involve the resident in planning for transfer. He or she is ultimately the decision-maker in the relocation.

Evidence suggests that ensuring continuity of care for elderly persons during care transitions improves patient outcomes, reducing the rate of avoidable rehospitalizations. Comprehensive discharge planning and transitional care also improve quality of life and satisfaction with care, and reduce individual patient costs by as much as 37% in one year.

The Bottom Line

Improving care as a means of reducing hospitalizations is sensible—depriving residents of needed care is not. All involved professionals must use good judgment and not lose sight of the resident's need for services. Some readmissions are not preventable and experts suggest that having some readmissions indicates the hospital provides quality care. What is certain is that readmissions are also the greatest avoidable cost that hospitals face. The readmission rate is listed as a quality indicator on the CMS Hospital Compare website. Refer to the Appendix of your book for a table listing facilities with the highest and lowest hospital readmission rates. Stephen Jencks, a healthcare consultant and former director of quality improvement at CMS, has stated that having a zero readmission rate "would be a very bad sign." Others note that providing financial incentives to keep people out of the hospital could cause hospitals:

- Not to readmit patients

- To discharge patients prematurely

- To discharge patients solely because they know they will receive less reimbursement (i.e., not for medical reasons)

Introspective long-term care personnel may wish to ponder the results of a study in the *Journal of the American Geriatric Society* that noted a "greater risk of multiple complicated transitions (bounce backs) in patients initially discharged to skilled nursing facilities" and "a lower risk of multiple complicated transitions for patients initially discharged to rehabilitation facilities" (Kind et al., 2007). This is a potentially thorny issue because private insurers and Medicare encourage residents who require rehabilitation services after a stroke, hip fracture, or joint replacement to transfer to an SNF instead of an inpatient rehabilitation facility (IRF). Taken at face value, the SNF is a cheaper alternative. The problem is that the bounce back factor is much greater in the SNF setting. For example, the rate of bounce back for a person with a joint replacement in an SNF is 14.3%. It is 2% to 3% in an IRF. If a person is admitted to an IRF after a cerebrovascular accident, he or she is three times more likely to go home compared with a person with similar problems admitted to an SNF.

Why Should I Care?

Saving Medicare dollars is everyone's problem. From a personal standpoint, you will need Medicare someday and it is important to ensure that our dwindling public resources last. From the facility standpoint, the census pays the bills. This includes the mortgage, utilities, food, and supplies. Salaries are the facility's greatest single expenditure. If the census decreases, staffing is likely to decrease, which will not make you happy. Raises will not be as generous or may be frozen entirely.

Facility survival

As nurses, we would like to believe that our services benefit humanity and that reimbursement is not an issue. However, we do not volunteer our time and most people work because they need a paycheck! We expect to be fairly compensated for the hours we work. The facility must generate an income to pay bills and meet the payroll. We prefer not to hear about census building, maintaining occupancy at or above the budgeted census, and other budget-related issues. Although these are not considered nursing functions, nurses have indirect control over them. These things are essential to meeting the payroll, keeping the lights on, ensuring quality care, and thus facility survival.

Keeping the lights on

Many workers believe that their salaries are the primary benefit received from the employer. You may not be aware of the intangible benefits that your employer provides. Although many frontline long-term care workers believe they are underpaid, researching the cost of your benefits can be enlightening. When you add up the employer's contribution to withholding taxes, sick pay, insurance, holiday pay, and numerous miscellaneous benefits, you may be surprised to find that the facility is actually paying twice your hourly wage for your services. The money to do this is generated by keeping the beds full. Recognizing this often helps workers develop a greater appreciation of the work environment and keeps the employer's contribution in perspective. One of the ways we ensure facility survival is by protecting the census and avoiding unnecessary hospital admissions and readmissions.

Where to Begin

Managing elderly residents with chronic illnesses is challenging. Residents of an SNF require close observation and attention to detail. Good communication, scrupulous care planning, identifying risk factors, anticipating and preventing complications, and coordinating care are essential services. With all these responsibilities, facilities must consider the causes of unnecessary readmissions and the many repercussions associated with rehospitalizations. Before transferring a resident, the nurse and physician should weigh the benefits versus risks and consider the potential for harm associated with transfer to another setting compared with the potential for benefit. Make the transfer only if the new setting will better meet the resident's needs. Facilities should have systems in place to prevent rehospitalizations. Goals and objectives should include:

- Accurate transfer of resident information from one facility to the next

- Healthcare professionals involved in the transition communicate appropriately before, during, and after the transfer

- Careful monitoring of residents who were recently admitted or readmitted after hospitalization

- Ensuring the transition is atraumatic for the resident and responsible party and is as smooth and seamless as possible for all parties

- Good coordination of facility services

- Being prepared to receive the resident by ensuring necessary drugs, equipment, and supplies are available

The information in this book will help you develop a plan to:

- Ensure transitions of care are fluid and coordinated

- Reduce avoidable rehospitalizations

- Reduce avoidable transitions

- Provide essential information to the resident's next care provider or setting

- Communicate clearly and appropriately both verbally and in writing about the resident and his or her needs

- Ensure that the transition is safe and satisfying to the resident

- Reduce costs associated with rehospitalizations

- Eliminate duplication of diagnostic services

- Decrease or eliminate the number of hospital observation stays (Chapter 5)

- Reduce the incidence of hospital readmissions resulting from avoidable complications, medication problems, and adverse events

- Encourage the resident and family to participate in the transition

- Ensure the resident and family express satisfaction with the care given in your facility

- Maintain or improve the resident's quality of life

Keep in mind that rehospitalization involves much more than paperwork errors. The hazards of readmission to the hospital include:

- Danger to residents

- Increased risk of errors, especially medication errors

- Disruption in the continuity of care

- Disruption in facility operations

- Economic viability of the healthcare system is affected

CHAPTER 2

Identifying the Origins and Causes of Problematic Transitions

Interfacility Communication

Good communication between providers increases the probability that a person will receive necessary care and education to meet his or her needs during the transition from hospital to long-term care facility (LTCF) (or vice versa). In fact, inadequate communication has been listed as a major factor for hospital readmissions. Hospitals blame LTCFs and LTCFs blame hospitals for inadequate communication and lack of information. Sometimes both parties misinterpret the Health Insurance Portability and Accountability Act (HIPAA) rules, believing the other party is not entitled to the resident's medical information. This further complicates a difficult situation.

LTCF Concerns

When information is missing, LTCF nurses have difficulty monitoring the resident's condition. Many LTCFs receive residents with:

- Incomplete or missing diagnoses

- No history and physical or discharge summary

- No advance directive information or code status

- Missing or incomplete medication lists

- No stop dates for time-limited orders such as antibiotics

- Missing lab and x-ray test results; no notification of significant tests with results pending

- No instructions for special procedures such as complex medical devices or wound care

- Lack of instructions and information for follow-up appointments, lab tests, and x-rays

- Orders that are unrealistic for the LTCF setting

- New infections and/or pressure ulcers

Physician Concerns

Another issue is that a hospitalist (a physician whose practice is devoted to treating patients in a hospital setting) or other specialist may care for the resident in the hospital. The treating physician has little or no contact with the facility attending. There is often no hand-off from one physician to another. Written records, discharge summaries, and diagnostic testing are often not sent to the attending who cares for the resident in the facility. Other issues include:

- The insurance may require a change of physician.

- The insurer may require hospital discharge before the person is ready.

- The medical director or other facility physician accepts the resident from another setting and is not familiar with the person's needs; little to no information is sent with the resident.

- The resident has dementia and/or is a poor historian. The attending physician is not familiar with the resident or her history.

- The physician phones a prescription to the pharmacy, such as a schedule II drug. The pharmacist advises the physician to fax the order. The physician is not in the office and has no access to a fax.

- Physicians are paid more for caring for patients in the hospital (refer to the chart in the appendix of your book). They fear their bills will be denied if they visit a LTCF resident more than once in 30 days.

  - The federal regulations specify that nursing home residents must be seen by a physician at least once (not only once) every 30 days for the first 90 days, then every 60 days thereafter.

  - Medicare does not limit physician visits to nursing facility residents as long as the visit is reasonable and necessary.

  - At times, some fiscal intermediaries have imposed arbitrary limits on payment for physician visits. A 2001 Institute of Medicine (IOM) report recommended removal of "arbitrary limits set by fiscal intermediaries on the number of [nursing home] visits." They noted that Medicare (and Medicaid) regulations for physicians' services in nursing homes should allow the number and type of services provided to be based on each resident's medical needs and the severity of their illness.

- It is easier for physicians to care for hospital patients. The doctor has a wide variety of diagnostics immediately available. He or she can make rounds and see a number of patients fairly quickly.

- Physicians are available 24 hours a day in the hospital to care for unstable patients and emergencies.

Schedule Drug Issues

Unfortunately, the inability to get schedule II drugs is a serious problem, especially on evenings, nights, and weekends. Toby S. Edelman, a senior policy lawyer at the Center for Medicare Advocacy, has stated, "If people are so sick that they desperately need pain medication, they should be seen by a doctor." Unfortunately, an after-hours visit is not likely to happen without sending the resident to the emergency department (ED). Even then, the person will get one dose and a prescription for a very limited supply of medication. The amount may be insufficient to cover an entire weekend. An ambulance (for which Medicare Part B pays the bill) will likely be used to transport the resident to and from the ED. The lack of in-house physicians has been a problem in LTCF for decades (Leland, 2010). The situation described here is a common one and is a huge waste of Medicare dollars.

The Drug Enforcement Administration permits hospital nurses to phone prescriptions for narcotics to the pharmacy. When phoning the drug orders to the pharmacist, the nurse is considered an agent of the physician. LTCF residents needing narcotic analgesics must suffer for 24 to 48 hours, or even longer, before receiving adequate pain relief. This is an unacceptable delay. The rules have been relaxed somewhat so facility nurses can phone in prescriptions for schedule IV narcotics, such as acetaminophen with codeine #3, and schedule III drugs, such as those containing hydrocodone. They cannot phone the pharmacy with orders for schedule II drugs such as morphine. Meeting this burdensome bureaucratic requirement causes avoidable pain that reduces quality of life, placing residents at risk for rehospitalization and violating quality of care standards. According to the American Medical Directors Association, a nursing facility physician writes an average of 169 prescriptions for controlled substances each month, leaving ample opportunities for delays (Leland, 2010).

Emergency Department Concerns

Most transfers from long-term care facilities to acute care hospitals go through the ED. On the hospital end of the spectrum, receiving personnel complain that some long-term care facilities send residents to the ED without the necessary information to provide treatment. The resident ends up taking a round trip ambulance ride from the LTCF to the ED and back. Residents are sometimes sent with no information, or poorly organized information that is of little value. ED personnel also complain that:

- Responsible party contact information is missing; the ED does not know if a family member has been notified of the transfer

- Advance directive information is not provided

- A list of medications is not furnished

- Allergy information is not provided

- The facility does not notify the ED of the resident's impending arrival and little information is sent with the resident

- The resident arrives at the ED with no information about the chief complaint or history of the present illness

- The resident is very unclean upon arrival at the ED

At the very least, the facility should provide the following:

- Diagnosis(es)

- Physician name

- Current problem/reason for transfer

- Most recent vital signs

- Past medical history

- Medications and allergies

- Baseline physical and mental status

- Advance directives

- Contact person at LTCF

- Telephone for contact person or responsible party

Patient and Caregiver Concerns

The factors identified by patients and caregivers to be most valuable to them during care transitions are:

- Assistance with medication self-management

- A medical information record owned and maintained by the patient to facilitate cross-site communication and information transfer

- An electronic medical record that can be accessed across care settings

- Timely follow up with primary or specialty care

- A list of signs and symptoms or warning signs suggesting a worsening condition and instructions on how to respond to them

Other factors that contribute to high rehospitalization rates are:

- Poor understanding and/or compliance with discharge instructions

- Lack of involvement of resident and family in discharge planning

- Lack of a current advance directive

- Physician lack of familiarity with resident and family wishes

- An unspoken facility or family preference for sending residents to the hospital to die

- Lack of a positive working relationship between facility nurses, residents' family members, and the attending physician

- Reluctance of nurses or family members to intervene when the physician makes a decision to hospitalize a resident

Surprising Information

You may be surprised to learn that LTCF residents with an acute infection who remain in the facility fare much better and have fewer complications compared with residents who are hospitalized for treatment (Boockvar et al., 2005). Overall, residents often fare better when they remain in the facility because:

- It is home and they are most comfortable in a familiar environment with familiar staff

- There is a reduced risk of relocation trauma

- Staff is familiar with the resident and is likely to identify changes from his or her "normal" quickly

CHAPTER 3

Reasons for Inappropriate Hospitalization and Rehospitalization

Most Common Causes of Inappropriate Rehospitalization

Many rehospitalizations are lengthier than the original hospitalization. The most common medical conditions requiring rehospitalization are:

- Heart failure

- Acute myocardial infarction

- Pneumonia

- Chronic obstructive pulmonary disease

- Psychosis

- Gastrointestinal problems

- Electrolyte imbalance

- Sepsis

The surgical procedures most likely to require rehospitalization are:

- Cardiac stent placement

- Percutaneous transluminal coronary angioplasty

- Coronary artery bypass graft surgery (heart bypass surgery)

- Major hip or knee surgery

- Vascular surgery

- Major bowel surgery

- Other hip or femur surgery

In addition to poor verbal and written communication described in Chapter 2, other factors that contribute to high rehospitalization rates are:

- Care plan from the discharging facility not communicated to the receiving facility

- Inadequate monitoring and supervision by discharging and/or receiving facility

- Inadequate follow-up care from long-term care providers

- Low hospital census

- Deterioration of a resident's condition

- Medical, nursing, medication errors, frequent medication switches, and adverse drug events

- Nursing or caregiver failure to notify the healthcare provider of changes in condition (in a timely manner)

- Physicians in discharging facility unwilling to write medication orders for residents who are cared for by a different physician in the receiving facility

- Facility turnover and staffing problems

- Pressure to admit residents to the long-term care facility (LTCF) in the evening and on weekends when there is less staff and a greater chance for error

- An acute exacerbation of a chronic disease

- Inaccurate or incomplete reporting from facility nurse to the physician

- A new problem that either developed in the hospital (e.g., a nosocomial infection, such as *Clostridium difficile* diarrhea), or was exacerbated by the hospitalization, such as a fall due to weakness and lack of activity in the hospital

- Necessary medications, supplies, and durable medical equipment not available

- The resident has not seen the primary caregiver since hospital discharge

- The resident is in an assisted living facility, which has fewer resources than other types of facilities

Financial Incentives

Some authorities suggest that LTCFs have financial incentives for sending residents to the hospital. The problem is that nurses on the units are the ones who have primary control over the transfer and most are not aware of the various methods of making money for the facility, nor do they care to do so. Although most LTCF nurses will disagree with the reasons listed here for transfer, a variety of sources believe they have merit. Common reasons are:

- If a facility sends a resident to the hospital, the resident often qualifies for skilled rehabilitation or Medicare skilled care (Chapter 5) upon return, which can be charged at a much higher rate.

- Facilities are paid Medicaid bed hold fees when residents are hospitalized. If the resident is not a Medicaid recipient, families and residents may also pay bed hold fees out of their private monies. Thus the facility collects money during the resident's absence but does not have to care for the resident.

Ending Hospital Readmissions: A Blueprint for SNFs

- Facilities are often paid bed hold fees for the resident's usual bed elsewhere in the facility when the resident is receiving services on a skilled (Medicare) unit.

- Another issue surrounds residents in the LTCF under the Medicare Part A (hospital insurance) payment plan (Chapter 5) in that the Medicare rate is all inclusive, meaning that the LTCF must use the Medicare payment to pay for drugs and most services the resident receives. Some residents are very costly. In fact, some facilities believe they are being underpaid for providing medically complex care. It is easy to see why a facility might have an incentive to send residents with expensive, acute conditions to the hospital for care.

Early Discharge

Many LTCF nurses complain that hospital patients are being discharged quicker and sicker. In 1969, the average length of stay (ALOS) was 10.6 days. However, patients age 65 and older stayed in the hospital an average of 14.2 days. By 1982, the ALOS had decreased to 10.1 days. Today the ALOS is only 6.4 days. Table 3.1 lists the average length of hospital stay over the years.

Early discharge from the hospital creates a great risk for rehospitalization. Reimbursement often drives care, and utilization review committees may try to discharge patients as soon as possible. Under the diagnosis-related groups (DRG) payment system, hospitals are paid a flat fee for the resident's stay. If the patient is discharged early, the hospital often makes money. If the person has an extended stay, the hospital loses money. Because of early hospital discharges, residents often require heavy care when they are admitted to the LTCF.

Discharging a resident too early also has a domino effect on the LTCF. Residents must meet certain criteria for Medicare to pay for their LTCF stay and payment is

| Table 3.1 | **Average Length of Hospital Stay** |

Year	Average Length of Stay
1940	13.7 days
1950	10.6 days
1969	9.3 days
1968	9.2 days
1970	8.0 days
1971	7.9 days
1973	7.8 days
1979	7.9 days
1980	7.5 days
1990	6.5 days
2000	4.9 days
2006	4.8 days
2009 (last year for which information is available)	4.6 days

time-limited. Medicare Part A (called hospital insurance) pays room and board for residents with qualifying conditions who have spent at least three consecutive midnights in the hospital. Many residents who would otherwise qualify for benefits in the skilled nursing facility (SNF) are disqualified because they have not had the qualifying stay due to early discharge. See Chapter 5 for additional information.

The Weekend Exodus

Some administrators dread returning to work on Monday after having the weekend off because facilities are often plagued with an epidemic of weekend hospitalizations, which have a devastating effect on the census. The "weekend exodus" involves discharging both new admissions and rehospitalizations. The administrator may apply pressure on the nursing department to try to reduce the rate of weekend hospital admissions, thereby maintaining the census. Some weekend hospitalizations are essential, but many are avoidable. Some reasons for the excessive hospitalizations are:

- The attending physician is not on call. The covering physician is unfamiliar with the resident and errs of the side of caution and orders hospitalization.

- Physicians who are not following the resident are reluctant to write orders.

- There is no physician on-site to evaluate sick residents; in order to be seen by a doctor the person must go to the emergency department.

- The attending physician is too far away or otherwise unable to travel to the facility in a timely manner, if at all.

- Physicians believe that Medicare auditors are more likely to question physician billing for frequent SNF visits, compared with hospital visits for residents who are acutely ill.

- Lack of availability of some diagnostic tests in the facility.

- Technology is not available to effectively diagnose and treat an acute event.

- Nursing staff are unable to provide skilled services needed by the resident.

- Notification of panic (critical) laboratory values.

- Treatment of abnormal laboratory values for conditions such as dehydration.

- Lack of coordination of care interfacility and intrafacility.

- Communication problems interfacility and intrafacility.

- Physicians prefer to treat residents in the hospital, where diagnostic tests, medications, and other necessities are readily available. Additionally, physicians receive higher payments for caring for hospital patients.

- Physicians and nurses fear legal exposure if a resident dies or experiences serious complications, especially if families insist on transferring a resident to the hospital and are overruled by the physician or a facility nurse.

- Some LTCF nurses are inexperienced or insecure about addressing the resident's medical problems and prefer to send the resident to the hospital.

- Staff are not trained or qualified to address the problem.

- Lack of advance planning, policy, and procedural resources.

- Inadequate medical resources.

- Short staffing, especially on weekends; staff feels overwhelmed.

Concerns about weekend hospital admissions

Lest you think that sending a resident to the hospital on a weekend is in the resident's best interest, consider this surprising information. A number of studies have revealed increased mortality on weekends and holidays:

- Five-day and 30-day postoperative mortality were significantly higher in patients admitted during holiday periods than during weekends and weekdays (Foss & Kehlet, 2006).

- Patients who are admitted to the hospital with acute kidney injuries are 22% more likely to die by day 3 of their stay if they are admitted during the weekend rather than on a weekday (James et al., 2010).

- Persons with end stage renal disease who are admitted to the hospital over a weekend are more likely to die earlier than those admitted on a weekday (Sakhuja, 2010).

- Survival rates from in-hospital cardiac arrest are lower during nights and weekends, even when adjusted for potentially confounding patient, event, and hospital characteristics (Peberdy et al., 2008).

- Patients admitted on weekends with a diagnosis of cerebrovascular accident had a 13% higher mortality rate (Saposnik, 2007).

- Weekend admission to an intensive care unit was associated with a significant increase in the risk of death (Ensminger et al, 2004; Kuijsten et al., 2010; Cavallazzi et al., 2010).

- Patients with abdominal aortic aneurysms (42% vs. 36%), acute epiglottitis (1.7% vs. 0.3%), and pulmonary embolism (13% vs. 11%) had higher weekend mortality in one study. In this study, differences in mortality persisted for all three diagnoses after adjustment for age, sex, and coexisting disorders (Bell & Redelmeier, 2001).

- Another study revealed that persons with pulmonary embolism who are admitted on weekends have significantly higher short-term mortality than those admitted on weekdays (Aujesky et al., 2009).

- A study of 230,000 patients who were admitted on weekends with a first heart attack had higher mortality rates at 30 days compared with those who were admitted on weekdays (Bell & Redelmeier, 2001).

- One team of researchers reported that patients with a first myocardial infarction admitted on a weekend had a 0.9% increase in mortality, or about nine to

10 additional deaths per 1,000 heart attack admissions. This could account for several thousand deaths each year in the United States (Bohan, 2007).

- Canadian researchers found that patients admitted on a weekend with a diagnosis of cerebrovascular accident had a 12% higher risk of dying than those who were admitted during the week, regardless of the severity of their condition. This is compared with a 7% death rate for patients admitted on a weekday. Although the reasons for the problem are unclear, the researchers suggested that having more staff on weekdays may explain the difference in death rates (McCook, 2010). Stroke is the third leading cause of death in the United States.

Some of the potential reasons for increased weekend mortality are:

- Severity of condition.

- Most patients who are admitted on weekends do so because of emergencies; most are not as medically stable as other patients.

- Increased alcohol, drug, and tobacco consumption on weekends.

- Reduced hospital staffing.

- Limited access to specialists.

- Unavailability of all services and invasive procedures.

- Lower use of procedures and lack of availability of specialized procedures over the weekend.

  - This may be related to the fact that most weekday procedures are scheduled in advance, but may also be an indicator of quality of care

- Specialists such as neurologists and interventional cardiologists are in the hospital on weekdays, but on call on weekends. Response time is much longer.

- Staff scheduled to work weekends may have less seniority and experience than those who work weekdays.

- Weekend staff are often relief personnel who are not as familiar with the patients as regular staff.

- Many facilities schedule fewer supervisors on weekends.

- Supervisors are often responsible for overseeing staff they do not know well and whose abilities and work routines are less familiar.

- Working weekends is less desirable, less staff are scheduled, and rate of call offs is higher.

- Further research is needed to identify accurate reasons for a higher weekend death rate.

Hospital discharges on Fridays

More hospital discharges occur on Friday than any other day of the week. One team of researchers found that patients discharged from the hospital on Fridays had an increased risk of death or nonelective rehospitalization within 30 days after discharge (van Walraven & Bell, 2002). Potential reasons are:

- The patients were less medically stable, but overly anxious to go home

- Discharges preparation were incomplete owing to competing demands on staff time due to multiple discharges on Fridays

- Hospitals try to discharge as many patients as possible because less staff is available on weekends

- Delays in implementing social services until the end of the week

The issue related to Friday discharges is also something to keep in mind. Further research is needed to identify why Friday discharges are associated with worse outcomes than discharges on other days of the week.

Medical Diagnoses and Conditions That May Predispose Residents to Acute Changes in Condition

Residents with some conditions are at higher risk for rapid, acute condition changes and instabilities. Residents with these diagnoses need regular monitoring, even if their conditions are stable. After hospitalization, frequent monitoring and targeted assessments are necessary to identify changes before the condition becomes acute. Consider listing special monitoring for potential problems on the care plans of residents with these conditions and diagnoses (refer to the examples in the Appendix of your book).

- Cardiopulmonary

  - Congestive heart failure

  - Hypertension

  - Myocardial infarction

  - Aneurysm

  - Acute exacerbation of chronic obstructive pulmonary disease

- Functional impairment or decline

  - Acute impairment of one or more activity of daily living (ADL)

  - Impaired mobility

  - Recurrent falls during past three months

- Prolonged bed rest

- Urinary retention

- Metabolic

  - Diabetes mellitus.

  - Malnutrition.

  - Dehydration, volume depletion, hypernatremia, hyponatremia, electrolyte imbalance.

  - Weight loss.

  - Endocrine disease.

  - Abnormal chemistry profile values.

  - Blood urea nitrogen (BUN) over 22 mg/dL.

  - Elevated sodium over 147 (suggests severe dehydration).

  - Elevated serum creatinine: A creatinine greater than 1.5 suggests renal disease. If elevated, determine the BUN/creatinine ratio. Divide the BUN by the creatinine. Values over 23 indicate dehydration.

- Hematocrit (greater than three times the hemoglobin)

- Potassium below 3.5, over 6

- Chloride over 107

- Glucose < 50 and > 300

  - Excellent guidelines for reporting laboratory values may be downloaded from *http://tinyurl.com/23ejy53*

- Additional information about panic values and other reportable laboratory values is available in the Appendix of your book

- Musculoskeletal

  - Muscle weakness secondary to old stroke

  - Osteoporosis

- Neurological

  - Pain

  - Cerebrovascular disease

  - Cerebrovascular accident

  - Transient ischemic attack

- Neuropsychiatric

  - Confusion

  - Depression

  - Dizziness, impaired balance

  - Mild/moderate dementia

- Sensory

  - Vision/hearing impairment

- Systemic/general

  - Postoperative status

  - Pressure ulcers

      – Polypharmacy; use of multiple medications (usually four or more daily)

      – Taking antibiotics

      – Taking anticoagulants

- Other

      – Cancer

      – Gastrointestinal disease

      – Presence of infection or an infectious disease

New Onset Problems Suggesting an Impending Change in Condition

In addition to abnormal vital signs and abnormalities detected during focused physical assessment, the following issues suggest an actual or potential acute change of condition and should be assessed further.

Behavioral symptoms

- Significant change in nature or pattern of usual behavior

- New onset of resistance to care

- Abrupt onset or progression of significant agitation or combative behavior

- Significant change in affect or mood

- New onset violent/destructive behaviors directed at self or others

Cognitive symptoms

Delirium is an acute confusional state that is commonly caused by medical illness. Signs and symptoms can be new onset problems such as confusion and untoward behavior in an alert resident or a worsening of confusion in a resident with existing cognitive impairment. Acute delirium is characterized by changes in behavior, reduced awareness of the environment, and disorientation. The most common causes of delirium are infectious, circulatory, respiratory, and metabolic disorders. Dehydration is a very common cause that usually responds to increased fluids if the problem is identified soon after the resident becomes symptomatic. Causative conditions can occur simultaneously or can aggravate existing dementia. Accurate diagnosis includes at least two of the following:

- Abrupt onset of or increase in confusion

- Memory impairment

- Reduced or fluctuating levels of consciousness

- Perceptual disturbances, including misinterpretations, hallucinations, paranoia, delusions, and illusions

- Change in psychomotor activity

- Insomnia and disturbance of sleep–wake cycle

Elimination patterns, change in

- New onset of frank blood in stool, urine, or vomit

- New onset coffee ground emesis

- Abrupt change in frequency of urination or defecation

- Frequent loose stools (three or more in 24 hours)

- New onset incontinence

- Worsening incontinence of bowel or bladder

Most Common Causes of Inappropriate Rehospitalization

Falls

- New onset of falls not attributable to a readily identifiable cause

- Recurrent falls over several days to several weeks

- More than one fall on the same day

- One or more falls with a subsequent change in neurological status or findings suggesting a possible head injury

Functional ability

- Sudden or persistent decline in function (i.e., ability to perform ADL and instrumental ADL)

Level of consciousness

- Distinguish the resident's level of consciousness (LOC) from other aspects of cognition such as orientation and memory. Levels of consciousness are:

  - Alert

  - Drowsy or lethargic

  - Stuporous

  - Comatose

- Changes that suggest a change in condition:

    - New onset fluctuation or deterioration in LOC

    - Alteration or frequent fluctuations in LOC

    - Reduction of one level or more in LOC (e.g., from alert to lethargic, or from lethargic to stuporous)

    - Lethargy, hypersomnolence (sleepier than usual or sleepy for most of the day)

Pain

- Pain worsening in severity, intensity, or duration and/or occurring in a new location

- New onset of pain not associated with trauma

- New onset of pain greater than 4 on a 10-point scale

Weakness

- New onset of weakness

    - Define/describe weakness as generalized or localized

    - Describe weakness in detail

Weight/eating patterns

- Abrupt change in appetite before a significant change in weight occurs

- Rapid weight gain or loss

- Significant weight gain or loss (5% in 30 days, 10% in 90 days)

- Change in meal intake pattern; eating 50% less than usual over past 24 hours

  - Document intake and fluid consumption in as much detail as possible

  - Consider intake and output

  - Initiate calorie count

- Change in fluid intake pattern; drinking 50% less than usual over past 24 hours

  - Document intake and fluid consumption in as much detail as possible

  - Consider intake and output

  - Initiate calorie count

- Signs and/or symptoms suggesting fluid imbalance (e.g., edema or change in edema)

  - Acute, rapid weight gain over several days

  - Acute, rapid weight loss over several days

CHAPTER 4

Risk Factors

Identifying Risk Factors

Identifying risk factors that may result in a change in condition and developing a preventive plan of care is an essential nursing responsibility. Residents who have recently been admitted or readmitted from the hospital have a number of risk factors. Surprisingly, one risk factor for rehospitalization is living in a long-term care facility (LTCF). Medicare recipients living in LTCFs have higher rates of emergency room visits and rehospitalizations than their peers in the community. This may be related to weakness and loss of function during hospitalization:

- 30% of all geriatric residents experience functional decline during hospitalization

- 50% of these residents return to their prior baseline function after returning to their usual residence

Also consider that:

- 20% to 40% of those over 65 are admitted to an LTCF at some point

- Skilled nursing facilities have an approximately 25% annual mortality rate

- 50% of those admitted to skilled nursing facilities require short-term postacute care and expect to return home at the time they initially enter the facility

- LTCF outcomes are highly dependent on function at admission

In order to reduce unnecessary hospital readmissions, facility nurses must be able to identify who is at risk. In addition to the high-risk medical and surgical diagnoses listed in Chapter 3, residents who are at high risk for readmission include:

- Elderly (age 65 and over)

- Male gender

- African American

- Cognitively impaired, depressed, or having mental health problems

- Persons who do not speak English

- Living in a rural area

- Living in a low income area

- Living in the south

- Residents who are relatively new to the facility and staff is not familiar with their medical problems, wishes, and preferences

- Having any of the following chronic conditions:

  – Diabetes

  – Respiratory conditions

  – Circulatory conditions

  – Dementia and behavior problems causing the resident to become aggressive with other residents or staff

Ending Hospital Readmissions: A Blueprint for SNFs

- Having any of the following acute conditions:

  - Dehydration

  - Bacterial pneumonia

  - Urinary tract infections

Another problem that contributes to unnecessary hospitalizations is that family members sometimes panic when residents with palliative care, hospice, and do not resuscitate (DNR) orders deteriorate. The facility has little choice but to comply if the family demands the resident be sent out.

Table 4.1 summarizes additional factors that contribute to rehospitalizations.

| Table 4.1 | | Factors Contributing to Rehospitalizations |

Systemic Factors	Clinical Factors	Resident and Family Factors
Long-Term Care Facility		
Available of resources in LTCF	Clinical diagnoses	Resident and family awareness of LTCF capabilities and ability
Sufficient personnel	Underlying disease	Weighs benefits versus risk of hospitalizing the resident
Good communication and collaboration	Physician confidence in ability to manage the residents' changing conditions	Lack of understanding and regular review of advance directives
Monitoring and assessment	Presence of complications	Personal preferences
Availability of diagnostic tests	Risk of complications	Provision of palliative care
Physician or other care provider availability	Clinical stability	Provision or use of hospice
Availability to provide IVs and advanced clinical services	Level of function	Confidence in hospital or LTCFs ability to provide services

| Table 4.1 | | **Factors Contributing to Rehospitalizations (cont.)** |

Systemic Factors	Clinical Factors	Resident and Family Factors
Long-Term Care Facility		
Ability to respond promptly to changes in condition	Degree of independence	Strain of frequent hospitalization on resident
Availability of supplies	Mental status	Relationship with physician and facility staff
Good communication with physicians and local hospitals	Nutritional state	Understanding of resident condition
Thorough assessment of residents prior to admission to ensure needs can be met	Adequacy of hydration	
Bed availability	Vital signs	
Bed hold policies and procedures	Physician or care provider visits	
Provision of Medicare skilled services	Physician or care provider communication with facility	
Medication availability	Availability of skilled nursing care	
Adherence to regulations	Problems and goals	
Hospital	Frequency of nursing assessment and monitoring	
Familiarity with local LTCFs	Medication administration	
Personnel knowledgeable and qualified to provide gerontologic care	Provision of treatments	
Availability of specialists	Diagnostic tests	
Ability to accurately identify and assess patient needs	Prognosis	
Bed availability in hospital		
Discharge planning should begin at time of admission		
Good communication with LTCF		
Availability of LTCF beds for discharge		

The tools for identifying rehospitalization risk have been developed for use by acute care hospitals. The Hospital Admission Risk Profile (Sager et al., 1996) is a simple tool that can be used by LTCFs to assess residents for risk of rehospitalization. It may be downloaded from *www.annalsoflongtermcare.com/images/43-44_ altc0409TryThis.pdf.* The Probability of Repeated Admission Research Summary is also a simple, useful tool that is widely used by LTCFs. This tool that is available from *http://tinyurl.com/23s87mh.*

The Polypharmacy Problem

Polypharmacy is the use of many drugs simultaneously. This is fairly common problem with elderly adults, including those residing in LTCFs. Although drugs provide many beneficial effects, the potential for polypharmacy is great. Consequences include:

- Adverse drug reactions

- Drug-to-drug interactions

- Noncompliance with the drug regimen

- Decline of quality of life or functional ability

- Deterioration in mental status

Polypharmacy information

- Elderly persons consume more medications than any other age group.

- Although 15% of the U.S. population is elderly, the over-65 age group uses approximately 30% of all prescription medications and 40% of the over-the-counter (OTC) drugs sold.

- Taking two drugs increases the risk of an adverse event by 6%. An elderly person taking six different drugs has an 80% risk of at least one drug–drug interaction. Taking eight medications increases the risk by 100%.

- Adverse drug events rank fifth among the top preventable health threats to elderly persons in the United States, after congestive heart failure, breast cancer, hypertension, and pneumonia.

- A study of hospital admissions revealed that polypharmacy and adverse drug events reactions were present in 10% to 12% of the patients admitted to a hospital medical service.

- In 2008, the FDA received more than 530,000 reports of adverse drug reactions. Of these 33,000 were submitted directly to the FDA, primarily by drug manufacturers. That same year, there were 320,000 serious adverse events and nearly 50,000 deaths.

- A large study of nursing home residents revealed that 31% experienced serious preventable adverse drug events. Another 56% had reactions that were deemed significant events. Failure to adequately monitor the residents was identified as the cause in 49% of the adverse events.

- A national study found that nursing home residents take an average of 6.7 routinely scheduled medications, plus up to 2.6 medications on an as needed basis. Twenty-seven percent of nursing facility residents take nine or more routinely scheduled medications.

- Drug interactions are a leading cause of adverse drug events.

Nursing action

Nurses should:

- Review the resident's drug regimen monthly or more often. Check for drugs with questionable purpose, taking two similar drugs to treat the same problem, inappropriate or incorrect dosages, and changes in the resident's condition that warrant a change in dosage or discontinuation of any medication.

- Review new drug orders carefully to ensure that adverse drug reactions are not being managed with additional medications.

- Review possible interactions between the medication regimen, herbs, vitamins, and OTC drugs the resident is taking.

- Monitor for drug-to-drug interactions. For example, interactions commonly occur between anticoagulants and nonsteroidal anti-inflammatory drugs (NSAID) or aspirin. If the resident uses NSAIDs regularly, avoid concurrent aspirin use.

  – Review and monitor the drug–drug interactions on the M3 drug list available on the downloads page

- When evaluating the drug regimen for potential drug interactions, include drugs that were recently discontinued. Drugs with long half-lives are cleared slowly, so the risk of interactions can last for a prolonged period of time. For example, drug interactions with fluoxetine (Prozac®) may develop as long as six weeks after it has been discontinued.

- Teach residents and paraprofessional staff (such as medication aides) common side effects and potential food and drug interactions to avoid.

- Teach residents and staff to report new symptoms that suggest an adverse drug reaction.

- Encourage fluids when giving medications. Water is a diluent for medications. Dosages are calculated by body weight and an assumed distribution of water in the body. Residents with less water in the body may have a higher concentration of drug per kilogram of body weight. Dehydrated residents readily experience drug toxicity.

- Each LTCF has a consultant pharmacist who is responsible for monthly reviews of each resident's medication regimen. If you have questions or concerns about a side effect, drug interaction, or need for regular blood level monitoring, contact your consultant promptly.

- Inform the physician if you believe a drug is causing an adverse effect. Document your notification, nursing action taken and the physician's response.

Medication Reconciliation

Medication reconciliation is a formal process of compiling the most current, complete list of a resident's medications, then using the list as a resource of accurate medications anywhere in the health system. An analysis of medication-related errors reported that 66% of reconciliation-related errors occurred during transitions. Of these, 22% occurred during admission and 12% at discharge. The most common errors were drug omissions and prescribing mistakes.

Nursing action

Medication reconciliation is required by The Joint Commission during care transitions. This applies to all accredited hospitals and LTCFs. However, it is a good practice in all facilities, including those that are not Joint Commission-accredited. Facilities should reconcile medications at admission, transfer, and discharge. The medication reconciliation process consists of:

- Obtaining original medication bottles, if possible, and documenting the resident's home medications on a single list

- Confirming the accuracy of the home medication list by questioning the resident or responsible party

- If the resident was admitted from the hospital, documenting the hospital medications on a separate list

- Comparing the home and hospital medication lists with the facility medication list

- Ensuring that discrepancies identified (i.e., omissions, modifications, deletions) are appropriate based on the resident's care plan

- Resolving unintended discrepancies with supporting documentation

- Communicating medication information during transitions in care

- Performing medication reconciliation at admission, readmission, transfer, and discharge

- Notifying the healthcare provider of discrepancies, changes, and omissions and verify whether the practitioner wishes to reorder any medications that were stopped during or after the resident's hospitalization

The Joint Commission suggests developing a medication reconciliation form for collecting medication information, standardizing care, and preventing errors. Joint Commission-accredited facilities are required to reconcile:

- Prescription medications

- Sample medications

- Vitamins

- Nutraceuticals

- OTC drugs

- Vaccines

- Diagnostic and contrast agents

- Radioactive materials

- Respiratory therapy-related medications

- Parenteral nutrition

- Blood derivatives

- Intravenous solutions (plain or with additives)

- Any product designated by the FDA as a drug

Refer to additional information in Chapter 8 and the appendix of your book. A comprehensive medication reconciliation toolkit may be downloaded from *www.ncqualitycenter.org/downloads/MRToolkit.pdf*. A good medication reconciliation training program is available at *www.nmh.org/nm/education+training*. You will find an example medication reconciliation policy in the appendix of your book. Forms may be downloaded from *http://tinyurl.com/37nl4rq* and *http://tinyurl.com/2dx9vea*. Free registration may be required.

The Patient Self-Determination Act

The Patient Self-Determination Act (PSDA) has been a federal law since 1991. The PSDA requires healthcare facilities and providers who receive federal Medicare or Medicaid funds to offer written information explaining each person's legal options for accepting or refusing treatment in the event they are incapacitated or at the end of life. The law ensures that persons entering healthcare facilities are given information about their right to execute an advance directive. The PSDA laws vary from state to state. The significant provisions of the federal act are:

- Hospitals, LTCFs, home healthcare agencies, hospices, and health maintenance organizations are required to maintain written policies and procedures guaranteeing clients written information explaining their involvement in treatment decisions. The facility must provide state-specific information and written policies of the facility regarding implementation of these rights. The medical record must contain documentation regarding whether the individual has implemented an advance directive. In general, the organization has no obligation to supply specific forms on which to document treatment decisions, although some do this.

- The healthcare facility employer must provide education for staff and the community regarding advance directives.

- Each state is required to develop written descriptions of the law concerning advance directives in their jurisdiction and provide this material to healthcare providers.

- An advance directive may be a living will, a durable power of attorney for healthcare, or both:

  - Durable power of attorney for healthcare gives a person of your choice the authority to make healthcare decisions for you in accordance with your wishes, including your religious and moral beliefs, if you are not capable of making sound decisions yourself. The designated person must follow your instructions. He or she may consent, refuse to consent, or withdraw consent to medical treatment and may make decisions about withdrawing or withholding life support. A physician and healthcare facility must comply with your agent's instructions or allow you to be transferred elsewhere. The agent's authority begins when a physician certifies that you lack the competence to make healthcare decisions. If your ability to make decisions returns, the decision-making power automatically reverts back to you. Thus, the durable power of attorney for healthcare may be a temporary or permanent appointment.

- A living will is a form that communicates your wishes about medical treatment in the event that you become unable to communicate them due to illness or injury. The living will is based on your beliefs, ethics, religion, and personal values. You may want to consider what burdens or hardships you would be willing to accept for the benefit obtained if you are seriously ill. A living will does not take effect until a physician certifies that you are terminally ill. In some states, two physicians must verify the terminal illness. When signing this document, you may specify the type of care you desire, whether it is aggressive, limited, or comfort care only.

• Some states have additional, state-specific forms, such as those used for out-of-hospital cardiac arrests, or a healthcare surrogate directive form for use when a critically ill person has not signed a directive and is incompetent or incapable of communication. In the long-term care setting, the resident may be given the opportunity to sign a directive upon admission. This is usually the social worker's responsibility, but in some facilities nurses provide the information. Many facilities will provide the forms, but are not legally obligated to do so. Facilities should not provide legal advice concerning advance directives. The resident or responsible party should be referred to their attorney for specific legal information. If the resident does not sign an advance directive upon admission, he or she may sign one at any time.

Nurses' responsibility

The American Nurses Association (ANA) published a statement describing the nurses' responsibilities in implementation of the PSDA. The ANA recommendations state that nurses should be familiar with the laws of the state in which they practice and should understand the strengths and limitations of each form of advance directive. For additional information and ANA position papers on a variety of subjects related to ethics, human rights, advance directives, resuscitation, and end of life care refer to *http://tinyurl.com/27jku3u*.

Special situations

Although all states have laws providing for designation of advance directives, the individuals who may witness the execution of directives vary from one state to the next. Become familiar with your state laws. In many states, nurses and nursing assistants directly caring for the person may not witness the document. Persons with a financial interest in the operation of the facility, such as the facility administrator, may be prevented from witnessing the form. The best option may be to ask another alert resident, a resident's family, or facility visitor to witness the signing of the document, unless this is prohibited by state law. Other issues to consider are:

- States regularly modify and change their advance directive forms. Because of this, you must carefully read the form the resident gives you. The language on the form signed by the resident may be different than it is today. The original form may be used. A new form is usually not necessary. Follow the instructions on the form signed by the resident.

- In most states, a caregiver who is not related to the person by blood or marriage may not be designated as the durable power of attorney for healthcare.

Physician's orders and facility policies

Keep a copy of the signed directive on the medical record. Give the original to the resident or responsible party. If the resident is transferred to the hospital or other healthcare agency, send a copy of the document with the transfer form. Inform the ambulance service and emergency department that the resident has a directive.

If the advance directive requests no cardiopulmonary resuscitation (CPR), you must obtain a physician order. Your state laws will specify the type of order needed, such as a DNR or "allow natural death" and many facilities require this order to be written in the physician's handwriting. Some will accept a phone order, but two nurses must witness the order. Follow your facility policy.

Nursing response

This is where things become confusing. Do not automatically assume that the presence of an advance directive means you must obtain a DNR order. Do the following:

- Read the directive. Make sure that withholding CPR is in keeping with the resident's wishes, as stated on the form.

- See if there is a statement on the directive that says something to this effect: "If, in the judgment of my physician, I am suffering with a terminal condition from which I am expected to die within six months, even with available life-sustaining treatment provided in accordance with prevailing standards of medical care."

- Find out how your facility policies define "life-sustaining care" or "heroic care." If the resident is not in terminal, irreversible condition, as certified by a physician, you should not withhold routine care or emergency care because of the presence of a DNR order.

- Review and become familiar with the language on the various advance directives used by your state, at various times from 1991 to date. Getting blanket DNR orders whenever the resident has a "no heroics" directive is not a good response and it may increase the legal vulnerability of the nurse and the facility.

Difficult situations

You may encounter some advance directive issues that need clarification:

- If your state law or advance directive form requires the physician to certify the resident as being in terminal condition, you will need further clarification. For example, if the resident with no known terminal illness chokes on food in the dining room, you should perform CPR. This is an accident/emergency that is unrelated to terminal illness. By getting a DNR order, are you depriving the resident of emergency care? In many facilities, the answer to this question is yes! Be careful and be sure you understand the proper action to take.

- Consider a resident who has no known terminal illness who becomes dehydrated and requires an IV and antibiotics for a serious urinary infection. If the resident has a DNR order, will you provide IV therapy, or is this considered life-sustaining treatment? In some facilities, IV therapy is withheld in the presence of a DNR order, whereas in others, an IV is considered routine care.

Revoking the advance directive

A resident can revoke an advance directive at any time. However, the laws for revoking a directive are less clear. Most commonly, a resident will verbally revoke the advance directive by telling the nurse of his or her wishes. Follow your state laws. Does your state permit you to witness the revocation? This could become a nasty legal issue if the resident verbally revokes the directive during the night and dies before morning. At the very least, the revocation should be in writing, if possible, and supported by the signature of the resident and two witnesses. The best approach is to be proactive. Learn your state laws regarding advance directives before you are in this position.

Advance directives have been an issue in numerous lawsuits filed by family members of LTCF residents. Some sue for wrongful life, whereas others sue for wrongful death. You may wish to review the legal opinions written for nurses in the Legal Eagle Eye archives at *www.nursinglaw.com/#step1*. Search keywords such as "advance directive," "code," "do not resuscitate," and "cardiac arrest." Know and follow your state laws and facility policies to protect yourself and your facility. State laws are always changing. Keep up with changes mandated by the legislature in your state. For additional information, you may wish to review "10 Legal Myths About Advance Medical Directives" at *www.pdcaregiver.org/10Myths.html*.

Why Is This Important?

Multiple rehospitalizations are common during the last six months of life. Many residents are sent to the hospital to die, usually via emergency ambulance. Consider a proactive stance that helps the resident face life's end and enables him or her to die in comfort, in familiar surroundings. Focus on advance care planning and resident and family education about advance directives, palliative care, and the use of hospice.

Hospice Care

The hospice philosophy involves:

- Affirming life and neither hastening or postponing death

- Supporting and caring for the resident in last phase of life so he or she can live as fully and comfortably as possible

- Providing holistic care to the resident, including physical, mental, social, and spiritual care

- Assisting the resident's family to cope

- Creating an environment that provides the resident and family members with satisfactory mental and spiritual preparation for death

- Maintaining function, relieving suffering, and optimizing quality of life

Medicare-qualified hospice admission criteria are:

- Life expectancy of less than six months

- The resident gives up all standard Medicare benefits

- The program must be a certified hospice program

- The resident must agree to forego curative care

Although the Medicare hospice benefit requires a terminal prognosis, Medicare recognizes that an exact date of death cannot be identified. As a result, residents and facilities are not penalized if hospice services exceed six months.

When a resident is admitted to hospice, the hospice provider assumes responsibility for managing the resident's care. However, because the resident is in an LTCF, two separate regulatory systems may be involved (one for hospice and one for the nursing facility). The rules that are presently in place remit two separate payments to the hospice. One payment is for the interdisciplinary professional management services provided by hospice personnel. The other payment is for room and board at 95% of the prevailing Medicaid nursing facility rate for the resident's bed. The hospice pays the LTCF for the resident's room and board and other basic services. The hospice provides medications and necessary supplies, such as a commode and therapeutic mattress. The Medicare-certified hospice and the nursing facility must have a formal contract because of the dual coverage situation. Services covered by the Medicare hospice benefit are:

- 24/7 on-call services by necessary hospice personnel, who are not required to be on location in the facility

- Physician services

- Nursing services

- Services of a home health aide

- Social services

- Physical, occupational, speech, and respiratory therapy

- Equipment and medical supplies required for palliation of illness

- Medications for symptom management and pain relief

- Short-term hospitalization/respite care

Although not specifically stated, most hospices also provide the services of other professionals, such as a dietitian and members of the clergy.

The hospice is technically responsible for the resident's care and the facility is expected to keep them informed of any and all changes in condition. The care plan must represent a joint effort between both organizations. The hospice must retain professional management responsibility for all contracted services. Certain essential services must be provided by hospice employees. Nonessential services may be provided by the facility. The hospice is required to have a written plan of care covering:

- Physician and nursing services

- Physical, occupational, speech, and respiratory therapy

- Medical social services

- Home health aides and homemakers

- Short-term inpatient care

- Counseling

- Respite care

- Medical supplies, drugs, and biologicals

The hospice situation is in flux as this book goes to press. This is a profitable type of care and facilities with hospice contracts should be aware that hospice enrollment decisions are being closely scrutinized with an eye for fraud and abuse. Medicare has considered changing the end of life care rules for residents in LTCFs. They have proposed paying LTCFs an additional fee to provide end of life care, with the option of contracting with hospice for consulting services only. However, no one is certain that the majority of nursing facilities are willing to assume this responsibility. If this proposal is enacted, one major change is that the resident would not be required to forego curative care.

Residents with dementia

The report of a study released in December 2010 revealed that more residents with dementia are using the Medicare hospice benefit and using it for longer periods of time than in the past, although there are state-by-state variations (Miller, 2010). This is significant because approximately 40% of LTCF residents die with some degree of dementia. The paper, published in the *American Journal of Alzheimer's Disease and Other*

Dementias, is the first to estimate the statistics for long-term care residents who die with mild to moderately severe or an advanced degree of dementia. This is an important indicator of the prevalence of dementia in the long-term care population.

Review the resident's advance directive and discuss his or her wishes for end-of-life care. Make a hospice referral, if acceptable to the resident and family. This will enable the resident to remain in the facility to face death with comfort and dignity.

CHAPTER 5

Medicare Part A Basics

The Medicare Program

Medicare is a federally funded program for elderly and disabled individuals that pays for certain services in the hospital, long-term care facility (LTCF), and home health-care settings. The four primary types of Medicare you may see in the LTCF are:

1. Medicare Part A: hospital insurance; pays for hospital and skilled nursing care.

2. Medicare Part B: medical insurance; there is a charge of approximately $100 a month for this coverage, which is deducted from the Social Security check. Some people have opted not to pay this premium, thus have no Part B coverage. Some people will pay $96.40 and others will pay $110.50 in Part B premiums in 2011, depending on income. The cost usually increases annually. Part B pays for laboratory work and x-rays, physician visits, some medical supplies, and therapy services three days a week.

3. Medicare Part C: Medicare Advantage; this is an optional service that some people have elected. Medicare pays a premium each month to insurance companies. These insurers cover the individuals. Medicare does not. Most, if not all, are managed care plans. As a rule, they offer many extra benefits at little to no cost. However, they are managed care plans and, as such, have complete control over the services the person receives. Many problems and hospitalizations require

preapproval. Preapprovals are not necessary with the original Medicare plan. Part C plans also specify health providers and hospitals where the beneficiary must go for service. This is an opt-in program. Medicare beneficiaries may elect to use the Part C program during open enrollment from October through December each year. Likewise, they may drop the Part C plan and return to the regular Medicare fee-for-service plan during the October to December open enrollment period.

4. Medicare Part D: the Medicare drug plan. Beneficiaries pay a premium for this annually, based on the plan they select. They usually pay for this by check or bank deduction. Some have it deducted from the Social Security check. They also pay a copayment for each prescription. Part D covers many, but not all, prescriptions until drugs reach a certain dollar amount.

5. Unless otherwise noted, the information in this chapter pertains only to Medicare Part A, hospital insurance.

Medicare spending

Ten percent of all Medicare beneficiaries account for 58% of all Medicare spending. This may result from elderly individuals with multiple chronic conditions and/or functional and cognitive limitations. (These data do not apply to the Medicare drug plan and those enrolled in Medicare Advantage plans.) About 3% of all Medicare beneficiaries live in LTCFs. These residents account for about 5% of all Medicare spending.

Hospitals are paid a flat rate for a patient's length of stay. Under this system, the payment for a patient is the same whether they stay two days or 10 days. There is obviously a great financial incentive to discharge patients as early as possible. Early discharge works well if the person returns home, but Medicare is now recouping part of the diagnosis-related group (DRG) payment if the person is admitted to a lower level of care. Needless to say, the system saves Medicare dollars, but hospitals are not happy with the reduced payment.

Medicare Part A coverage, copays, and length of hospital stay

Some individuals pay a premium each month for private supplemental "Medigap" insurance to cover copayments and costs Medicare does not cover. These policies may be purchased only within the first six months of Medicare coverage. Beneficiaries cannot elect to purchase them at will. This type of policy will pay only if Medicare pays first. In order to qualify for Medicare coverage, a hospital stay must be considered both reasonable and necessary. The Medicare program is confusing at best. Lack of understanding of the Medicare program is a primary reason that residents and their responsible parties do not protest early hospital discharges. Many do not realize that they have a right to appeal.

PACT DRGs

In 1997, Medicare instituted the 10 pilot postacute care transfer DRGs (PACT DRGs). The payment varied for these diagnoses based on the DRG and its geometric mean length of stay (GMLOS). If the hospital discharged a patient to a lower level of care, such as home health or long-term care, hospital payment was reduced if the patient did not remain in the hospital for the full length of stay for the DRG. This was done because Medicare believed they were paying twice for that person's care if the full DRG was not used. Payment #1 went to the hospital and payment #2 went to the subsequent facility or agency. As a result, Medicare developed a reduced payment methodology for persons with PACT DRGs that were discharged early. A listing of all Postacute and Special Post-acute MS-DRGs (Table 5 of the IPPS Final Rule) is available at *http://tinyurl.com/49yfway*.

The new payment system worked so well that Medicare has expanded the list of PACT DRGs each year. For 2007–2008, approximately 37% of the 745 total Medicare DRGs were in the PACT DRG category. When the patient has a PACT DRG diagnosis, the patient must meet one of these discharge criteria:

- Discharged to a hospital or hospital unit that was excluded from payment under the prospective payment system

Ending Hospital Readmissions: A Blueprint for SNFs

- Discharged to a skilled nursing facility (SNF)

- Discharged to home but with a written care plan for home health services with the home care services being related to the reason for which the person was hospitalized; the home health services must be started within three days of discharge from the acute care hospital

This has little to do with operations in the LTCF other than some potential notations in the common working (billing) file, but this writer does not want to leave you with the misimpression that Medicare hospital care is pure profit. Medicare Part A is not always a profitable venture. What we do know is that our incoming residents are sicker and much more dependent than in years past. Today's residents are not "walkie-talkies." Most are heavily dependent and require a high level of care at the time of admission. Table 5.1 lists the most common diagnoses in the over-65 age group.

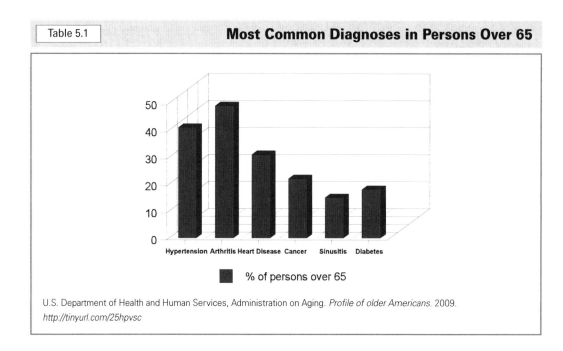

| Table 5.1 | **Most Common Diagnoses in Persons Over 65** |

U.S. Department of Health and Human Services, Administration on Aging. *Profile of older Americans.* 2009. *http://tinyurl.com/25hpvsc*

Ending Hospital Readmissions: A Blueprint for SNFs

Observational Hospital Admissions

Many patients are staying in the hospital under observational status, which is an out-patient service category. This means they are not formally admitted or considered inpatients. These individuals are usually too sick to go home or return to the LTCF. However, the hospital believes they are not sick enough to require "acute care," despite the fact that they are occupying a bed on a regular acute care hospital unit. Very few observational patients are aware that they are in the hospital under outpatient "observational" status. They just know they are in the hospital. This further complicates a confusing situation. Admission under observational status is also more expensive for the patient compared with inpatient care.

The physician is responsible for deciding whether his or her patient should be admitted as an inpatient. However, a chart review often reveals that the medical records of Medicare beneficiaries have no formal physician order for admission. Many physicians do not specify the type of care, leaving this up to the hospital to make the determination. Inpatients and outpatients are cared for on the same unit and the physician is not always aware of the patients' admission categories.

Use of observational status used to be rare, but has become a routine practice in the past few years. Hospitals are paid less for observational stays than they are for full admissions. Recent data reveal that claims for observation care rose from 828,000 in 2006 to more than 1.1 million in 2009. Claims for observation care lasting more than 48 hours tripled to 83,183.

Medicare began a pilot program in six states several years ago. Auditors are evaluating hospital utilization of services. Most hospitals fear being penalized for having too many admissions or readmissions. Patients in observational status are technically not admitted. This reduces the risk of federal scrutiny and penalties.

Ending Hospital Readmissions: A Blueprint for SNFs

This issue has nothing to do with "greedy" insurers limiting coverage. They do not get commissions or extra money for denying claims. The Medicare fiscal intermediaries (FI) are insurance companies. Centers for Medicare & Medicaid Services (CMS) is shifting responsibility for claims processing to new entities known as Medicare administrative contractors (MACs). The FIs and MACs make coverage decisions based on the "reasonable and necessary" Medicare criteria. This process is changing due to the Medicare Modernization Act (MMA). By 2011, the 23 fiscal intermediaries and 17 carriers will be replaced by 23 MACs, which will process both provider and institutional claims. Four additional MACs will process claims for durable medical equipment (DME) providers.

Much of the claims processing is done electronically, using software developed by CMS, but determining medical necessity may require a manual review. The MAC may request additional information to support the claim. Other computerized edits are done to identify fraud and abuse and ensure that the CMS billing policies are followed. Each intermediary and MAC have a medical advisor who also makes decisions and helps set policy.

After the claims review, the MACs issue the checks. The money is paid from a bank account funded by the Medicare trust fund. The amount of payment is based on national fee schedules, geographic adjustments, provider characteristics, and copayment requirements.

The FIs and MACs are paid according to the number of claims they process, regardless of whether the claims are accepted or denied. After the claims are paid, the MACs randomly select additional claims for further review. Medicare covers about 99% of the procedures and items submitted for payment. In 2008, Medicare paid the insurers $1.08 billion for processing 970 million claims from doctors, hospitals, and other healthcare providers.

Medicare auditors subsequently visit facilities and do random, on-site audits. These auditors are paid commissions for identifying hospital overcharges. This would occur if an auditor identifies patients who were admitted under inpatient status instead of observation. If the auditor finds the admission was not reasonable and necessary, the hospital must reimburse Medicare. They will also pay hefty fines. In extreme cases, overcharging Medicare can be prosecuted as fraud. Most facilities did not overcharge deliberately. Many of the problems were due to improper coding. During the three-year pilot project, noted above, facilities were required to return $1 billion in improper payments. The program was expanded to all 50 states in 2010.

Persons admitted under observation status are often those with conditions the hospital fears will be denied Medicare payment. Claims for observational care are usually paid without question. As a rule, hospitals are not usually penalized for admitting patients under observational status. Unfortunately, being an observational admission disqualifies the person from using Medicare-reimbursed skilled nursing care benefits after hospital discharge.

Medicare requires that patients whose status is downgraded from inpatient care to observation must be informed. Many are not notified. However, even if the patients are notified, most do not grasp the ramifications of this change in status. Patients have few appeal options or grounds for changing to inpatient care even if they know they are observation patients. Medicare is paying for their care on an outpatient basis, so benefits have not been refused. This eliminates their appeal rights. Refer to the additional information on the Medicare payment chart in the Appendix of your book.

Medicare generally expects patients will remain in observation status for no more than 24 to 48 hours. However, there are no time limits, so some patients spend longer periods of time in observation. The typical hospital response is that 48 hours is an arbitrary period of time and that discharging some patients at the 48 hour time

Ending Hospital Readmissions: A Blueprint for SNFs

limit would be inappropriate. The patient remains on observation status and is not considered an inpatient despite the longer stay. It should be noted that Medicare can deny payment for observational stays, but this is rarely done. However, the rate of denials has increased over the past few years. If Medicare denies payment, the patient becomes responsible for the entire bill.

A three-day hospital stay could actually consist of one observation day plus two inpatient admission days, or any combination thereof. This does not meet the qualifying stay requirement for SNF admission. Unless questioned specifically, some hospital discharge planners are anxious to move patients out quickly and are not forthcoming in providing the SNF with this information at the time of hospital discharge. If the SNF is not made aware of the observational admission status, they may admit the resident under the Medicare program. An excerpt from Medicare's description of observational status is provided in Table 5.2.

Implications of observational hospital admissions

In addition to being more expensive for patients, overusing observational days in the hospital has the potential for increasing rehospitalizations. Those who are unexpectedly discharged, have had inadequate discharge teaching, or do not understand after care instructions are also likely to return to the hospital, as are those who are medically fragile and unable to care for themselves at home.

Table 5.2	**Medicare Observation Status**

Observation services are defined by Medicare as a set of specific, clinically appropriate hospital outpatient services, which include ongoing short-term treatment, assessment, and reassessment before a decision can be made regarding whether patients require further treatment as hospital inpatients or if they are able to be discharged from the hospital. CMS expects that, in the majority of cases, the decision whether to admit a patient for inpatient services or discharge the patient can be made in less than 48 hours, usually in less than 24 hours. Only in rare and exceptional circumstances would it be reasonable and necessary for outpatient observation services to span more than 48 hours.

Observation care of more than 24 hours can have tremendous impact on Medicare beneficiaries. For example, Medicare beneficiaries are liable for approximately 20% of the costs of outpatient services that are paid by the Medicare Part B program while the patient is receiving observation and, in some situations, the full costs of self-administered drugs provided during that time. Further, a beneficiary must stay in the hospital a minimum of 3 days as an inpatient before Medicare will pay for SNF care; prolonged outpatient encounters do not count towards this statutory requirement.

*Excerpted from Richard Umbdenstock Medicare Observation Letter. July 7, 2010. Available at *www. hospitalmedicine.org/AM/pdf/menu-id-213.pdf*.

Medicare Paperwork in the Hospital

Hospitals are required to give patients a form entitled "An Important Message From Medicare – Your Rights While You Are A Medicare Hospital Patient" upon admission. This important document describes admission, discharge, and appeal rights. Unfortunately, patients are usually given many papers on admission. They seldom read them and are usually not aware of the importance of the Medicare paperwork. Some hospitals know this and take advantage of this fact. They can save money by ignoring the Medicare rules. Other hospitals do not have solid Medicare knowledge. They may not know that different rules and paperwork apply to Medicare patients or ensure their staff is properly trained. Either way, chances of being caught are slim. Medicare provides services to elderly persons and disabled individuals under age 65. Few of these individuals have a solid working knowledge of the complex Medicare rules. Teach your residents and responsible parties about using the Medicare system. Knowing how the system works is essential to receiving optimal care.

Notice of noncoverage

Most patients are not aware that Medicare rules have a provision to keep patients from being discharged from the hospital too soon. Knowing and applying this provision of the law is one way of ensuring a person meets the qualifying stay requirements for Medicare admission in an LTCF. A patient cannot be discharged until three days after the hospital gives the patient (or responsible party) a form called a "Notice of Noncoverage." The hospital cannot charge the patient who elects to stay for the full three days. If the hospital does not provide the notice, the three-day clock does not begin until they do. If the patient exceeds the three days, he or she is responsible for the bill. The cost can be substantial. However, many of the noncoverage decisions are reversed during the full appeals process. Even if the appeal is denied, the patient wins the battle although he or she loses the war. Filing the appeal often buys enough time to meet the qualifying stay and become eligible for LTCF Medicare benefits. The Medicare appeals process is confusing at best, but all Medicare beneficiaries have appeal rights. Additional information can be found at *www.medicareadvocacy.org*.

Inpatient Medicare Coverage and the SNF

Residents must meet certain criteria for Medicare to pay for their LTCF stay, and payment is time-limited. Medicare Part A (called hospital insurance) pays room and board for residents with qualifying conditions who have spent at least three consecutive midnights in the hospital. Upon facility admission, the resident may remain on Medicare for up to 100 days per spell of illness if he or she needs a daily skilled service or observation. To qualify:

- The resident must meet the three-day (three midnights) qualifying stay requirement

  - It is important to understand that the person must be fully admitted (not in outpatient observational care) and remain in the hospital for three midnights. This is because Medicare does not pay for the day of discharge. By staying for three midnights, the qualifying stay is met.

  - Services must be furnished in the most economical setting possible.

  - Services must be reasonable and necessary.

Unfortunately, there are no uniform definitions of "reasonable and necessary." In the past, the CMS have tried to define reasonable and necessary, but criticism and comments from various parties have thwarted the effort. Several lawsuits have tried to force this definition, but judges have ruled that CMS is not required to define the terms because the criteria are interpretive, making them exempt from federal rule-making requirements.

- "Reasonable" usually refers to the fee charged for the stay, treatment, or procedure. From our nursing perspective this is not relevant and outside of our control.

- "Necessary" refers to whether or not the treatment was necessitated by the condition for which the resident was hospitalized during the qualifying stay. This is proven by ensuring the resident has an appropriate diagnosis for every medication and treatment.

History of the three-day qualifying stay

The three-day rule was written in 1966 and is now obsolete, although it is still in effect. No one envisioned how things would change after the turn of the century. When the rule was written, Congress feared that families would admit loved ones to the hospital solely as a way of qualifying for 100 days of nursing home coverage. By gaming the system in this manner, the patient or family would potentially save thousands of dollars. The three days (three midnights) of medically necessary care were written into the rules as a means of preventing financial abuse of the system. Congress has given the CMS the authority to end the three-day rule, but only if this does not increase the cost. As you can see, nothing has changed and it is not likely that the three-day rule will be eliminated anytime soon.

Patients who do not meet the three-day (three midnights) inpatient qualifying hospital stay do not qualify for Medicare coverage in an SNF or other postacute care facility. Most facilities bill Medicare monthly. Residents who do not have the three-day qualifying stay will have their SNF Medicare billing denied. By the time the billing is done and the facility is notified of the denial, a substantial amount of money is lost. If the facility is aware of the observation status and denies Medicare coverage on admission, this often results in a very unhappy resident and family. The LTCF is almost always blamed for denying coverage, when they have no control over the length or type of hospital admission. Beginning an admission with an unhappy resident sometimes sets the tone for the entire stay.

As you can see, it is essential for the LTCF to verify the qualifying hospital stay. Technically, the person is not admitted to the hospital when "observation days" or "emergency room" (ER) stays are billed. Your bookkeeper may be able to access the billing information electronically by accessing the common working file (CWF) for your geographic region. Medicare beneficiary information is stored in the CWF. The CMS have divided the country into nine regions. Each has a MAC, who maintains the beneficiary claim records for the region. When a claim is processed, information is transmitted to the CWF. The CWF looks for beneficiary's records and processes the information. You should be able to use this information to determine whether the hospital stay is being billed as three full inpatient days or whether a combination of observation and ER days were also used. The CWF may also be used to check for possible duplication of services.

Medicare Level of Care and the LTCF

By definition, Medicare coverage is considered skilled, which is a higher level of care than required by most facility residents. Because of early hospital discharges, residents often require heavy care when they are admitted to the LTCF. Residents are assessed within five to eight days of admission with the minimum data set (MDS). Medicare assessments are repeated on the 5th, 14th, 30th, 60th, and 90th days (Table 5.3).

| Table 5.3 | | **Medicare Part A: MDS Assessment Dates** | |

MDS	Covered Stay Days (MDS sets payment for these days)	Assessment Reference Date (ARD)*	Grace Days Available
5 day	Days 1–14	1–5	3
14 day	Days 15–30	11–14	5**
60 day	Days 61–90	50–59	5
90 day	Days 91–100	80–89	5

*For Medicare Part A purposes, the assessment reference date (ARD) is used to identify assessments. This is the date listed at A2300 on the MDS. The ARD is the last day staff can collect information for the listed assessment. Changes that are identified after this date cannot be included. In other words, the ARD assessment accurately reflects the resident's condition. The ARD determines the coverage period of each assessment.

**If the 5-day assessment includes the CAAs and care plan, and is intended for use as the comprehensive assessment, the facility may use 5 grace days in which to complete the 14-day assessment. This does not apply if the comprehensive assessment (with CAAs and care plan) is not completed until day 14.

Under the Medicare program, the MDS is used to establish payment to the facility, based on a system called resource utilization groups (RUGs). (It is actually called RUG-IV, because the current system is version four.) "Utilization" is the term used to describe how much resource is used to care for the resident. The payment to the facility is determined by the medical services and functional support the resident is expected to need. RUG-IV consists of 66 groups divided into 16 categories (two were added) versus 53 under RUG-III. Each category has an established daily payment rate that is based on the estimated average amount of staff time, supplies, and services used. The average daily rate is $431.71 under RUG-IV. Rates range from approximately $130 a day to almost $700 a day. You should be aware that the Office of Inspector General issued a position paper entitled "Questionable Billing by Skilled Nursing Facilities" in December 2010. This document indicates that some facilities are placing residents into higher RUG groups than necessary, resulting in higher payment to the facility. This is an area that will be closely scrutinized in 2011 and beyond. A copy of this paper may be downloaded from *http://oig.hhs.gov/oei/reports/oei-09-99-00550.pdf.*

The first 20 days of admission are paid at 100% of the facility's Medicare RUG fee. From days 21 through 100, the resident must pay a substantial daily copayment. Medicaid covers the copayment fee for eligible low income residents. The Medicare payment to the facility serves as reimbursement for:

- Time

  - Nursing (RN, LPN/LVN, nursing assistants)

  - Rehab (OT, PT, SLP, assistants, aides)

- Nonrehab ancillaries

  - Medical supplies

  - Medications

- Lab

- Respiratory therapy

- Radiology

- General services

  - Building and grounds maintenance

  - Dietary

  - Laundry

  - Activities

  - Capital expenditures

  - Buildings

  - Equipment

The facility must also reimburse contracted outside entities for Medicare-covered services that are subject to consolidated billing. Excluded services that can be billed to Medicare Part B (medical insurance) include most physicians' services, emergency services, and ambulance trips relating to the transport of a beneficiary from the LTCF to a Medicare participating hospital for an inpatient admission. The LTCF must pay for ambulance transports to or from a diagnostic or therapeutic site other than a hospital or renal dialysis facility.

All-inclusive fee

The Medicare daily fee paid for the care of each resident is an all-inclusive fee. This means that the facility is expected to pay for drugs, treatments, laboratory tests, medical supplies and equipment, and all other expenses related to the resident's care.

With few exceptions (i.e., beauty shop, cable television), the facility cannot bill separately for these services as they would with a private pay resident. Because the Medicare rate is higher, the copayment for days 21 through 100 may also be higher than the facility's private pay fee. This is because residents who pay privately pay separate bills for their medications and all other services. While the resident is on Medicare Part A copayment, the fee remains all-inclusive. It is important that private pay residents understand this concept because the tendency is to refuse the Medicare coverage at day 21 because of the cost. The copayment may well save the resident money by limiting charges for which he or she would normally pay under the usual private pay rate. Someone with a sound understanding of the Medicare program must explain this to the resident or responsible party.

Many facilities fear Medicare denials, so they discharge residents immediately after day 20 as a matter of course. This way, there are no problems collecting copayments from Medicaid and others and Medicare is not likely to deny payment for claims lasting 20 days or less. Some facilities have had problems with denials beginning with day 21. The average Medicare-covered nursing home stay in 2007 was about 27 days.

Another wrench in the works is that many hospital skilled units admit residents for 20 days, then discharge them to the nursing facility. The first 20 days are fully covered and there is no copay. Claims are seldom questioned or denied during the first 20 days. When the hospital uses days 1 through 20, the resident returns (or is admitted) to the LTCF at a time when denials are likely. Some facilities will not run the risk of admitting the resident under the Medicare program after day 20, for fear of denial. The resident ends up losing. A few more weeks of coverage could mean the difference between life in a facility and returning home.

The problem with this situation is that many of the residents who are discharged at day 20 often need more skilled care and truly qualify for more Medicare coverage.

However, facilities may be unwilling or unable to take the risk. Our job as nursing personnel is to understand the reimbursement system well enough to find a way of advocating for the resident and legitimately continuing coverage. The coverage is often there, but a solid working knowledge of the Medicare rules is needed to identify it. We must also ensure that our documentation supports the need for this coverage. The Medicare program pays two to three times more for rehabilitative services than Medicaid does for long-term care services. Because of this, some facilities have expanded their rehabilitation programs to attract residents with Medicare benefits to offset losses related to inadequate Medicaid reimbursements. Earning this extra money enables the facility to continue providing high quality care. In addition to direct care, the higher level of care required for residents using Medicare observational care and care plan management calls for a higher level of assessment and nursing time with the resident. Spending this extra time with the resident increases the odds that you will identify and manage changes in condition early, before rehospitalization becomes necessary.

Spell of illness

The Medicare program pays for 100 days per spell of illness. This is a source of great confusion for facilities and an important concept to understand:

- There is no limit to the number of spells of illness for each resident; and

- The resident does not have to use all 100 inpatient Medicare days before beginning a new spell of illness

A spell of illness begins with the first day of Medicare-covered (SNF) care in the facility and ends (is broken) when the resident is either:

- Discharged for 60 consecutive days; or

- Does not require skilled care (according to the Medicare criteria) for 60 consecutive days

Ending Hospital Readmissions: A Blueprint for SNFs

Example 1: Mr. Strong is admitted for skilled therapy after a hip fracture. He has no other skilled services. Mr. Strong is discharged from Medicare on day 21. There are 80 days remaining in this spell of illness, but he does not use them. He does well and eventually returns to his former level of function. He remains in the facility. A year later, Mr. Strong is hospitalized for pneumonia. When he returns to the facility, he is in a new spell of illness with 100 days of Medicare coverage. The spell of illness begins again with a new 100 days. It does not pick up the 80 unused days. His first 20 days of readmission should be billed at the full Medicare rate, with no copays.

Example 2: Mrs. Wojciewski is admitted with a gastrostomy tube feeding. She is skilled because she receives more than 26% of her caloric intake and 501 mL fluid or more per day via tube. She cannot administer her own feeding, so uses all 100 days of Medicare coverage. She also remains in the facility and continues to receive a gastrostomy feeding. A year later, she is hospitalized for a severe urinary tract infection. Because she had the continuous tube feeding (which Medicare considers a skilled service), she has not broken the spell of illness. She has no Medicare coverage when she returns to the facility. In order to break the spell of illness, she would:

- Have to go home (with a family caregiver) for 60 consecutive days, or

- Not require tube feeding for 60 consecutive days, or

- Take less than 26% of her caloric nutrition and less than 501 mL of fluid per day by tube for 60 consecutive days. (A tube feeding comprising 26% of the caloric intake and 501 mL fluid or more per day is a skilled service. Less than that is not.)

Day of discharge and bed holds

As with the hospital, Medicare does not pay for the day of LTCF discharge if the resident returns home. There is no provision for Medicare payment of a bed hold if the resident is hospitalized or during a leave of absence in which Medicare require-ments are not met. In 2008, the rules were changed to permit the resident to pay privately for a bed hold, if desired. This is not to say that residents must remain in the facility at all times. Medicare permits therapeutic passes during times when Medicare services are not being given.

Lawsuits

If the resident receives a judgment or jury award as a result of a lawsuit related to his or her Medicare-covered condition, the resident is expected to repay Medicare and Medicaid (and also most private insurers) out of the proceeds of any damage awards received as a result of litigation. Many individuals are not aware of the repayment provisions of the law.

Other Important Reimbursement Issues

Beginning in 2008, Medicare stopped paying hospitals for preventable complications that were not present on the patient's admission. These events are formally called hospital-acquired conditions (HAC) or informally called "never events." CMS defines never events as "serious and costly errors in the provision of health care services that should never happen." This category includes errors such as wrong body part surgery, or mismatched blood transfusions, and others that cause serious injury or death. Additional information can be found in the Appendix of your book

The primary goals of this change in Medicare coverage were to:

- Reduce errors

- Improve patient care

- Give hospitals a financial incentive to prevent "never conditions" from occurring

Reducing deaths due to preventable medical errors and saving money were secondary objectives. A 1999 study revealed that medical errors cause almost 100,000 deaths each year and cost more than $29 billion annually. Medicare pays hospitals approximately $110 billion annually. They predicted that an estimated savings of $21 million annually would be realized by refusing to pay for the approximately 500,000 procedures necessary to correct never events. As this book goes to press, the list of complications for which hospitals will not be paid includes:

- Wrong body part surgery

- Wrong patient surgery

- Wrong surgery or procedure on a patient

- Foreign object retained after surgery

- Air embolism

- Blood incompatibility

- Pressure ulcers, stages III and IV

  - Stage I and II pressure ulcers and ulcers that developed and subsequently healed during hospitalization are not penalized

- Falls and trauma resulting in:

  - Fracture

  - Dislocation

  - Intracranial injury

  - Crushing injury

- Burns

- Electric shock

• Catheter-associated urinary tract infections

• Vascular catheter-associated infection

• Manifestations of poor glycemic control, including:

- Diabetic ketoacidosis

- Nonketotic hyperosmolar coma

- Hypoglycemic coma

- Secondary diabetes with ketoacidosis

- Secondary diabetes with hyperosmolarity

• Surgical site infection

• Mediastinitis following coronary artery bypass graft

• Surgical site infection following certain orthopedic procedures

- Spine

- Neck

- Shoulder

- Elbow

• Surgical site infection following bariatric surgery for obesity

• Laparoscopic gastric bypass

- Gastroenterostomy

- Laparoscopic gastric restrictive surgery

- Deep vein thrombosis and pulmonary embolism following certain orthopedic procedures:

    - Total knee replacement

    - Hip replacement

You may be surprised to learn that four never events also comprise 12.2% of total healthcare professional liability costs:

- Infections

- Injuries

- Objects left in the body during surgery

- Pressure ulcers

When Medicare patients are found to have allegedly preventable conditions at discharge that were not reported at admission, CMS reimburses the hospital only for the principal diagnosis at admission. Conditions that are present on admission are present at the time the order for inpatient admission is given. Conditions that develop in outpatient settings, such as the emergency department, observation, or outpatient surgery, are considered present on admission as they occurred prior to inpatient admission.

At the time of this writing, the HAC payment pertains only to hospitals for inpatient stays. Nursing facility payments have not changed. This is important to know because you may accept a person with an HAC, such as a pressure ulcer. The facility will be paid for caring for the resident.

Impact of never conditions

Some experts predict that hospitals might begin to avoid high-risk patients as a result of loss of revenue. Some believe that there are no completely effective approaches for preventing infection and some of the other listed conditions. They speculate that some conditions are present but not identified at the time of admission. (This makes a case for accurate documentation of admission and discharge assessments at both the hospital and LTCF. If the hospital disputes an HAC, it is conceivable that the nursing facility records will be audited.) Some experts question whether infections are 100% preventable and whether asking hospitals to prevent them is fair. Some state that pressure ulcers are caused by poor circulation and that the best nursing care cannot prevent them if the person's circulation is poor. This group of dissenters has been quite verbal about their belief that it is not fair or productive to penalize hospitals for the presence of HAC conditions. Other experts have proposed alternative approaches and incentives for reducing adverse events. At this time there is no consensus on how to do it better.

Critics say that the do-not-pay policies have been ineffective in improving quality, lowering cost, and reducing these conditions and have asked payers to try some new approaches. In July 2010, CMS reported that HAC policy yielded a net savings of $18.8 million for fiscal year 2009.

What to do

At the time of admission or transfer to the hospital, carefully document whether a resident has any of the conditions covered by the HAC program. Careful initial assessment and documentation of the never conditions will protect the facility. You may also consider working with your facility's quality improvement organization (QIO) to develop best practices and improve outcomes. You will find a complete list of QIOs in the Appendix of your book.

Ending Hospital Readmissions: A Blueprint for SNFs

Trendsetting

Medicare has always been a trendsetter and the never conditions are no exception. The Department of Health and Human Services secretary is to report to Congress by January 1, 2012, whether this policy should apply to other Medicare providers. A number of private payers, including Aetna, Wellpoint, Cigna, and seven Blue Cross Blue Shield associations, have already followed suit and ceased never event reimbursement, although each has developed their own list of do-not-pay conditions. Beginning on July 1, 2011, several private insurers and the Medicaid program will stop paying for preventable conditions acquired in hospitals and LTCFs. How this will shake out in practice is unclear. The law specifies that payment will be cut to states and not providers. The statute requires that the regulations "shall ensure that the prohibition on payment for health care-acquired conditions shall not result in a loss of access to care or services for Medicaid beneficiaries," although it is unclear what this means in that payment cuts are mandated.

The Patient Protection and Affordable Care Act (health reform legislation), passed in 2010, introduces the "Hospital Readmissions Reduction Program" that will affect Medicare payments. Beginning on or after October 1, 2012, Medicare payments to hospitals will be reduced if a hospital experiences "excessive" readmissions. This term has yet to be defined. (Planned readmissions are exempted under this program.) Additional conditions may be added to the readmission list beginning in 2015. The important part is that hospitals with excessive readmissions for specified conditions will receive reduced payments for all inpatient discharges. Payment reduction will not be limited to discharges relating to excessive rehospitalizations. The incidence of hospital readmissions will be publicly reported on the Hospital Compare website.

As you can see, the development of avoidable complications is a significant issue that all healthcare providers must address to avoid a loss of reimbursement and improve quality of care. Further information, resources, regulations, educational resources, and links are available at *www.cms.gov/HospitalAcqCond*.

Documentation

Remember that your documentation supports reimbursement. Meaningful and complete documentation is essential with residents in the facility under Medicare Part A. Residents who are in the LTCF under the Medicare payment program must have a notation on the medical record related to their Medicare qualifying condition at least once every 24 hours. Most facilities require an assessment of the resident's skilled condition and needs and documentation each shift. These residents are skilled and most change often enough to require a notation one or more times each shift. Unfortunately, another reason facilities give for establishing an "every shift" documentation policy is related to documentation skips, which is a problem that plagues many LTCFs. If a note is required once in 24 hours, and the nurse gets busy, forgets, or otherwise fails to write this note, there is no documentation for the 24-hour period. Thus, most facilities require a note each shift, even if the resident is stable. Remember that the note should reflect the nursing assessment related to the resident's Medicare-covered condition. Your documentation should be objective. Avoid notes such as "call light within reach," "doing well," and "will continue to monitor." If you document an abnormal observation, state the nursing action you took as a result of the observation.

CHAPTER 6

Strategies to Avoid Rehospitalization for Caregivers

Avoidable Readmissions to the Hospital

In addition to causing unnecessary Medicare expenditures, elders in our culture prefer to live independently for as long as possible. They want a stable residence. Most want to avoid relocation. Those with sensory deficits have great difficulty changing environments. Many elderly persons develop delirium when the environment changes. Involuntary relocation may lead to physical or psychological declines, including death.

The purpose of this book is to address avoidable and unnecessary rehospitalizations, not all rehospitalizations. Long-term care nurses must use good judgment in monitoring residents. Avoid trying to deter necessary admissions. Always err on the side of caution and resident safety and remember that all hospital admissions are not preventable. Identify and address resident risk factors to prevent a worsening of condition. Monitor residents carefully.

Strategies for Reducing Avoidable Readmissions

There are a number of different situations and approaches to prevent rehospitalizations. Some things depend on the resident's situation. Others are determined by whether you are a staff nurse, charge nurse, or nurse manager. Some things are determined by facility operations, policies, and procedures. Yet others are influenced by the preferences and opinions of residents' family members. Another issue is that as nurses we work at the behest of physicians. When a resident has a change in condition, we often speak with a nurse in the physician's office, who relays the information to the physician. More often than not, the nurse instructs us to send the resident to the emergency department (ED, ER), after which he or she is admitted. It is essential that we ensure our communication is clear. We also need to develop practices and protocols to address the resident's problems before sending them to the ER. The information in this chapter applies to staff and charge nurses who are on the front lines of resident care.

Improved transitions

Physicians, nurses, and social workers say better management of transitions to and from the hospital would minimize complications that result from a lack of adequate written and verbal communication, which sometimes result in preventable readmissions. Using the physician notification form in the Appendix of your book will help ensure that you communicate sufficient information for the physician to make medical and transition decisions. Set a goal that you will conscientiously manage transitions to and from the hospital and other facilities. Additional suggestions are:

- Remember, your goal is to prevent only avoidable readmissions, not all readmissions. Some rehospitalizations will be necessary. Never compromise a resident's welfare or safety. Err on the side of caution.

- When residents are admitted or readmitted, be sure to obtain complete physician orders, including code/no code.

  - Perform medication reconciliation at the time of each resident's admission and discharge.

  - For new admissions, obtain a complete and accurate list of each resident's current and preadmission medications, including name, dosage, frequency, and route.

  - If the resident was previously in the facility, reconcile medication orders with previous orders; clarify discrepancies. If the resident was at home, compare them with the home medication orders.

- If you are responsible for completing admission assessments such as pressure ulcer risk and fall risk, you are responsible for doing something with the information. These assessments are not done for paper compliance or personal edification. Once risk factors have been identified, nurses are responsible for planning care to reduce the risk and prevent adverse events.

- Teach all staff (including nursing assistants) about the rehospitalization problem and the need to prevent unnecessary readmissions.

- Give nursing assistants a complete report and instructions for residents who need monitoring. Advise them what to watch for. Avoid assuming they will identify abnormalities without direction and instruction. Question them about their findings periodically during the shift.

- Monitor residents who are not acting as they usually do and those who are known to be ill every two to four hours, or as needed according to your professional judgment.

- Monitor residents carefully for the condition for which they were hospitalized (or complications of this condition). (Refer to the documentation information and survey audit in the Chapter 7 Appendix of your book.)

  - Do a focused assessment every two to four hours, or as needed according to your professional judgment.

- Place a list of things to monitor on the front of the chart. (Refer to the examples in the Chapter 7 Appendix of your book.)

  - Lists of assessment points and documentation are available in *Clinical Documentation: An Essential Guide for Long Term Care Nurses*, which can be purchased at *www.hcmarketplace.com/prod 4923.html*.

Ending Hospital Readmissions: A Blueprint for SNFs

- Use the care plan! Keep it up-to-date. Report from it! It is more than paper compliance!

- Include the need for regular monitoring on the plan of care.

- Analyze stages of the care delivery process for strengths and weaknesses; address weaknesses.

- Develop a plan of action for individual residents to reduce unnecessary rehospitalizations:

  - List the plan on the care plan.

  - This involves careful monitoring and regular focused assessments.

- Evaluate and prioritize improvement opportunities.

- Monitor your unit's progress.

- Teach residents and families about the need to prevent avoidable readmissions.

- Monitor for the drug interactions in Table 6.1.

- Provide a holistic, resident-centered approach to care that encourages, allows, and engages the residents and families in the process of transfers, values that input, and facilitates their decisions. A knowledgeable resident can be an invaluable partner in care.

- Encourage independence to the greatest extent possible throughout the resident's stay. Provide restorative nursing. A resident who is dependent will be unprepared to assume responsibility for self care at the time of discharge.

- Use the forms and tools in the Appendix of your book for monitoring, reporting, and documentation.

| Table 6.1 | The M3 Project: Top Ten List |

Statistically, if a resident takes six different drugs, he or she has an 80% chance of at least one drug–drug interaction. The Multidisciplinary Medication Management (M3) Project has developed a list of 10 drug interactions that are particularly problematic in long-term care settings. Each of the drug combinations listed has the potential to cause significant harm if not managed appropriately. Medications chosen for the Top Ten list were based on their frequency of use in older adults in the long-term care setting and on the potential for adverse consequences if used together. The drugs and drug interactions on the Top Ten list are listed here.

Drug Interaction	Drugs in This Category
Warfarin—NSAIDs*	Aleve, Anaprox, Anaprox DS, Ansaid, Arthrotec, Cataflam, Clinoril, Coumadin, Daypro, diclofenac, diclofenac/mistoprostrol, diflunisal, Dolobid, etodolac, Feldene, flurbiprofen, ibuprofen, Indocin, Indocin SR, indomethacin, ketoprofen, ketorolac, Lodine, Lodine XL, mefenamic acid, meloxican, Mobic, Motrin, nabumetone, Naprelan, Naprosyn, naproxen, Orudis, Oruvail, oxaprozin, piroxicam, Ponsel, Relafen, sulindac, Tolectin, Tolectin DS, tolmetin, Toradol, Voltaren, Voltaren XR, warfarin
Warfarin—Sulfa drugs	Bactrim DS, Bactrim SS, Cotrim DS, Cotrim SS, Coumadin, erythromycin/sulfisoxazole, Gantanol, Gantrisin, Pediazole, Septra DS, Sulfatrim, sulfamethizole, sulfamethoxazole, sulfisoxazole, Thiosulfil Forte, trimethoprim/sulfamethoxazole, warfarin
Warfarin—Macrolides	azithromycin, Biaxin, clarithromycin, Coumadin Dynabac, dirithromycin, E-Mycin, erythromycin base, EES, erythromycin ethyl succinate, Ery-Tab, Eryc, EryPed, Erythrocin, erythromycin stearate, Ilosone, erythromycin estolate, Pediazole, erythromycin/sulfisoxazole, Tao, troleandomycin, warfarin, Zithromax
Warfarin—Quinolones**	alatrofloxacin, Avelox, Cipro, ciprofloxacin, Coumadin, enoxacin, Floxin, gatifloxacin, Levaquin, levofloxacin, lomefloxacin, Maxaquin, moxifloxacin, Noroxin, norfloxacin, ofloxacin, Penetrex, sparfloxacin, Tequin, trovafloxacin, Trovan, Trovan IV, warfarin, Zagam
Warfarin—Phenytoin	Coumadin, Dilantin, phenytoin, warfarin

Ending Hospital Readmissions: A Blueprint for SNFs

Table 6.1	The M3 Project: Top Ten List (cont.)

Drug Interaction	Drugs in This Category
ACE inhibitors – Potassium supplements	Ace Inhibitors - Accupril, Aceon, Altace, benazepril, Capoten, captopril, enalapril, fosinopril, lisinopril, Lotensin, Mavik, moexipril, Monopril, perindopril, Prinivil, quinapril, ramipril, trandolapril, Univasc, Vasotec, Zestril
	Potassium supplements - K+ Care ET, Kaon, K-dur, Klor-Con, K-Phos, Micro-K, potassium acetate, potassium acid phosphate, potassium bicarbonate, potassium chloride, potassium citrate, potassium gluconate, Urocit-K
ACE inhibitors – Spironolactone	ACE inhibitors - Accupril, Aceon, Altace, benazepril, Capoten, captopril, enalapril, fosinopril, lisinopril, Lotensin, Mavik, moexipril, Monopril, perindopril, Prinivil, quinapril, ramipril, trandolapril, Univasc, Vasotec, Zestril
	Spironolactone - Aldactone, spironolactone
Digoxin – Amiodarone	Digoxin - digoxin, Lanoxin
	Amiodarone - amiodarone, Cordarone
Digoxin – Verapamil	Digoxin - digoxin, Lanoxin
	Verapamil - Calan, Calan SR, Covera-HS, Isoptin, Isoptin SR, verapamil, Verelan
Theophylline – Quinolones**	Theophylline - aminophylline, Choledyl SA, oxtriphylline, Phyllocontin, Slo-Bid, Slo-Phyllin, Slo-Phyllin 125, Theo-24, Theo-Dur, Theolair, theophylline, Uniphyl, Uniphyl CR
	Quinolones - alatrofloxacin, Avelox, Cipro, ciprofloxacin, enoxacin, Floxin, gatifloxacin, Levaquin, levofloxacin, lomefloxacin, Maxaquin, moxifloxacin, Noroxin, norfloxacin, ofloxacin, Penetrex, sparfloxacin, Tequin, trovafloxacin, Trovan, Trovan IV, Zagam

*NSAID class does not include COX-2 inhibitors.
**Quinolones that interact include: ciprofloxacin, enoxacin, norfloxacin, and ofloxacin.
ACE, angiotensin-converting enzyme; NSAID, nonsteriodal anti-inflammatory drug.
Courtesy of Multidisciplinary Medication Management Project: *www.scoup.net/M3Project/topten.*

Standard of Care for Monitoring Residents With Acute Illness or Infection

All professions have standards for their members. The standard of care (standard of practice) is the degree of care or competence that one is expected to exercise in a particular situation. Standards represent minimum competencies for safe practice. Failure to provide care that meets or exceeds the established standards may cause resident harm and is cause for disciplinary action against the licensee. The standard of care is what a reasonable, prudent nurse would do in a given situation based on their education, experience, institutional policies and procedures, standards set by their professional organization(s), licensure board, regulatory agencies, textbooks, research, and professional literature.

Many individual standards apply to the care of each resident. The standard of care is not what the best professional would do, but rather what any reasonable professional with like qualifications would do in the same or similar circumstances. If a professional holds certifications and advanced education, he or she is held to the same standard as other professionals with similar qualifications. For example, if a nurse holds a certification in gerontologic nursing care, he or she is held to a higher standard than nurses without this certification. Review the information about long-term care standards in Table 6.2.

Table 6.2	**Standard of Care**

Each resident must receive and the facility must provide the necessary care and services to attain or maintain the highest practicable physical, mental, and psychosocial well-being, in accordance with the comprehensive assessment and plan of care. "Highest practicable" is defined as the highest level of functioning and well-being possible, limited only by the individual's presenting functional status and potential for improvement or reduced rate of functional decline. Highest practicable is determined through the comprehensive interdisciplinary resident assessment and by competently and thoroughly addressing the physical, mental, or psychosocial needs of the individual. The facility must ensure that the resident obtains optimal improvement or does not deteriorate within the limits of the right to refuse treatment and within the limits of recognized pathology and the normal aging process. When a resident shows signs of decline, surveyors will review the record to determine whether the decline is unavoidable. A physician statement that the decline is unavoidable will be considered, but is not accepted at face value without a detailed investigation of the situation. An accurate determination of unavoidable decline or failure to reach highest practicable well-being may be made only if all of the following are present:

- An accurate and complete assessment

- An assessment-based care plan that has been consistently implemented

- The resident's response to care has been evaluated and the care plan revised as necessary

From: §483.25 State Operations Manual

Close and careful monitoring and documentation that meet or exceed the standard of care are essential to identifying and preventing complications that lead to readmission to the hospital. Nurses and nursing assistants are responsible for regular and ongoing monitoring of residents who have experienced an acute illness, infection, incident, or other event. Any change in condition, even if minor, falls into this category. Monitoring continues for as long as necessary to ensure the event is resolved and the resident's condition has been stabilized. Most facilities monitor residents with problems or abnormal conditions at least once each shift until 24 hours after the condition is stabilized and the event resolved. In some situations, such as fever or head injuries, more frequent monitoring is required. If abnormal observations are noted, the nurse must take the appropriate nursing action, providing the necessary interventions and notifications.

If a resident experiences a change in condition, nursing personnel should:

- Use standardized risk assessments for every admission. Use the information to develop a plan of care to reduce the incidence of risk factors before the resident develops new complications.

- Monitor the resident regularly on all shifts until at least 24 hours after the acute event is completely resolved. Monitoring may continue for days or weeks, depending on the nature of the precipitating occurrence, and resident's response.

- Monitor residents every four to eight hours (every shift) for the first 72 hours of admission. Monitoring should include vital signs and focused assessment.

  - This should be a holistic process, not strictly a clinical assessment.

- Monitor vital signs (temperature, pulse, respirations, and blood pressure) at least once every eight-hour shift. Pulse oximetry may also be indicated. Check vital signs more frequently if one or more of the values are abnormal or the resident's condition warrants.

- Conduct a focused assessment of resident systems, based on the nature of the resident's problem at least once each shift. For example, for a resident with upper respiratory infection, the nurse should assess and document:

  - Auscultation of lung sounds. Assess the nature of sounds and adequacy of chest expansion, rate, rhythm, depth of respirations, and use of accessory respiratory muscles.

  - Vital signs (may be needed every four hours, depending on resident condition).

  - Pulse oximeter (may be needed continuously, depending on resident condition).

  - Color of the resident's skin, lips, and fingernail beds.

  - Change in mental status or level of consciousness.

Ending Hospital Readmissions: A Blueprint for SNFs

    – Increased restlessness.

    – Shortness of breath or other difficulty breathing.

    – Presence or absence of cough; if present, note if productive or nonproductive, with color, character, and amount of secretions. Describe condition of pharynx and complaints of sore throat, if any.

    – Presence or absence of signs and symptoms related to the specific infection; for example, presence or absence of nasal drainage.

- Report results of monitoring to the oncoming nurse in the change of shift report.

- Notify the physician immediately if abnormalities are noted. (Refer to the reporting guidelines in the Appendix of your book.)

- Inform the responsible party of the change and action taken.

- Update the care plan to reflect the additional observations, monitoring and care required because of the acute illness, infection, change in condition, or abnormal observation.

- Consider developing or using clinical (critical) pathways or care maps. Your facility can develop pathways and care maps specific to the setting or use some of the many excellent resources that are available online. Good sources of pathways are:

    – *www.carepathways.com/providers.cfm*

    – *http://tinyurl.com/257ce7w*

    – *http://tinyurl.com/22o8gqy*

    – *www.aapmr.org/hpl/clinpath.htm*

    – *http://tinyurl.com/2fwqrbu*

- Good sources of care maps are:

  – *http://caremapsforseniors.ca*

  – *www.snjourney.com/ClinicalInfo/CarePlans/CarePlanN.htm*

- Accurately and objectively document the results of monitoring, observations, nursing interventions, notifications, and the resident's response in the nurses' notes. If the resident is on antibiotics or other therapy, document the condition for which the antibiotics are being given. Avoid entries such as "no side effects to antibiotics." This is an appropriate entry in addition to other information, but absence of side effects can be easily noted on the medication record or flow sheet. Your nursing notes should address your assessment of the acute medical problem or injury and actions taken, as noted previously.

- If the resident is not responding to treatment for an acute medical problem, contact the physician.

- Identify the cause(s) of the acute change of condition and determine whether the resident can be managed in the facility.

Initial Assessment and Documentation Guidelines for Conditions for Which Monitoring Is Required

Assess and document the following every shift:

- Focused assessment on systems/problems with signs and symptoms of acute illness.

- Identify the resident's actual problems and/or complaints, if possible.

- Identify conditions that are unstable, or may become unstable.

- If the results of an assessment are positive, describe the nursing action taken.

Nursing action must be taken on positive assessment findings. Assessments with no action make both the nurse and the facility legally vulnerable and place the resident at risk. (Example: Assessment reveals crackles in lungs. Nursing action: contact healthcare provider, vital signs, increase fluids to liquefy secretions, encourage coughing and deep breathing, etc.)

- Describe negative findings. (Example: No chest pain, no cyanosis.)

- Document vital signs. If abnormal, describe nursing action taken.

- Initiate pulse oximetry.

- Determine if the abnormal findings are chronic or acute.

- Check for and consider recent laboratory values, if any.

- Evaluate the effects of new medications and side effects, if any.

- Monitor for signs and symptoms of inadequate fluid intake and dehydration.

  – Consider intake and output monitoring

  – Dehydration and inadequate fluid intake complicate many conditions

- Note any other changes from resident's usual condition (what he or she is like on a normal day).

- Determine whether other residents in the facility are being treated or have recently experienced the same or similar signs and symptoms.

- Consider whether a relationship exists between a current sign or symptom and a new medication, food or fluid intake, a change in activities, change in physical or mental condition, etc.

Specific Responsibilities

The specific roles and responsibilities in monitoring residents with acute change in condition include the following:

- Nursing assistant:

  - Recognize and report condition changes

  - Frequently observe the residents' conditions, symptoms, and vital signs

  - The offgoing nurse should review resident status with oncoming nursing assistants

  - Inform findings to a nurse and request follow-up nursing action

  - Inform a nurse manager if nursing follow up does not occur

- Staff nurse

  - Recognize changes in condition early

  - Assess the resident's symptoms, mental status, and physical function

  - Concisely document descriptions of observations and symptoms and nursing response

  - Update a charge or supervisory nurse if the resident's condition declines or does not improve within an expected period of time

  - Report the resident's status to the healthcare practitioner, as appropriate

- Charge nurse

  - Ensure residents are monitored consistently

 – Ensure residents are assessed accurately, in a timely manner

 – Review and evaluate documentation and reporting of relevant information

 – Ensure relevant information is communicated to other members of the
   interdisciplinary team with responsibility for the resident's care

- Attending physician/Primary healthcare practitioner

 – Respond to telephone notifications

 – Ask sufficient questions to arrive at a tentative diagnosis and develop a plan
   for initial workup and treatment

 – Ensure interventions are consistent with resident's advance directives

 – Communicate with the responsible party to discuss change in advance
   directives if the resident fails to improve as expected

 – Visit resident as needed

 – Avoid assuming that no news is good news

 – Remain in phone contact periodically until the resident's condition stabilizes

 – Communicate with other practitioners involved in the resident's care
   as needed

Mandatory documenting and reporting

The following signs and/or symptoms may be present to a greater or lesser extent if
an abnormality with any body system is present. The presence of these conditions
warrants an initial nursing assessment, reporting to the healthcare provider,
documentation of findings and notifications, and ongoing monitoring until
condition is stabilized.

- Pulse rate below 60 or above 100

- Pulse irregular, weak, or bounding

- Blood pressure below 100/60 or above 140/90, unless this is usual for resident

- Unable to hear blood pressure or palpate pulse

- Pain over center, left, or right chest

- Chest pain that radiates to shoulder, neck, jaw, or arm

- Shortness of breath, dyspnea, or any abnormal respirations

- Headache, dizziness, weakness, paralysis, vomiting

- Cold, blue, gray, cyanotic, or mottled appearance

  - Blue color of lips or nail beds, mucous membranes

- Cold, blue, numb, painful feet or hands

- Feeling faint or lightheaded, losing consciousness

- Respiratory rate below 12 or above 20

- Irregular respirations

- Noisy, labored, respirations

- Dyspnea, struggling, gasping for breath

- Cheyne-Stokes respirations

- Wheezing

- Retractions

- Blood sugar over 300

- Blood sugar less than 60

- Prothrombin time greater than 1.5 times the control value

- Sodium over 147

- Blood urea nitrogen (BUN) over 22

- White blood cell count over 11,000

- Hematocrit greater than three times the hemoglobin value

- Potassium below 3.5 or over 5.0

- Chloride over 107

- Elevated serum creatinine

  - A creatinine greater than 1.5 suggests renal disease. If elevated, determine the BUN/creatinine ratio. Divide the BUN by the creatinine. Values over 23 indicate dehydration.

Change of Condition Communication

Good communication skills are essential for observing changes of resident conditions and reporting them to the correct person.

- Document all communication with others regarding the resident.

- If a change in a resident's condition warrants physician notification, communicate essential information in a clear and logical manner that expedites understanding and intervention. Have all essential data available before making the call. Be direct and paint a word picture for the physician. Document his or her response. Complete the "Systems Check for Physician Calls" in the Appendix of your book to ensure you are focused and have complete information before contacting the physician.

- On weekends or during second and third shifts, you may communicate with an on-call physician instead of the attending. He or she may not be familiar with the resident. Clearly summarize the resident's background before describing the problem. Document his or her response.

- Document all attempts to reach the physician. If you observe significant or serious changes in a resident's condition, do not just chart them. Notify the physician. If he or she does not respond, notify the alternate physician, on call physician, or medical director. If the situation appears emergent, consider sending the resident to the emergency department by using facility standing orders, as permitted.

- Inform the responsible party of the initial change and keep him or her updated on resident response to treatment.

- Document notifications and referrals, such as notifying the social worker of the need for behavioral intervention, or the dietitian for a pressure ulcer, weight loss, or abnormal lab values.

- When obtaining physician orders for medications, you must also obtain a diagnosis to correspond with the medication. State the reason the medication is being given. Many medications have multiple uses.

- If the physician orders subsequent laboratory monitoring, make sure the lab is scheduled for the correct day and time.

- Legally, you must advocate for the residents. If you have reservations about the physician's orders, act on them! If, in your professional judgment, you believe the physician orders place a resident in jeopardy, you must intervene and clarify the treatment plan. If the physician is nonresponsive, contact your supervisor and go up the chain of command from there. Document the actions taken to advocate for the resident.

Interact II

The Interact II program has a number of resources and excellent tools, pocket cards, and reporting guidelines for frontline personnel to use in improving care and reducing avoidable hospital admissions. Several of these tools are appropriate for use by nursing assistants and other staff who have resident contact. Refer to *http://interact.geriu.org*.

CHAPTER 7

Strategies to Avoid Rehospitalization for Managers

Managerial Information for Reducing Acute Care Transfers

A collaborative approach and excellent communication are essential to reducing hospital readmissions. Residents are sometimes discharged from both the hospital and long-term care facility (LTCF) without adequate transfer information. Residents may be admitted to the LTCF without an adequate assessment of the resident's needs and a determination of the facility's ability to meet these needs.

Facility Admissions and Readmissions

The following facts and figures will help you recognize the scope and magnitude of the rehospitalization problem and its relationship to the LTCF:

- 40% of Medicare beneficiaries are discharged to a postacute care setting (LTCF, skilled nursing facility [SNF], home care, hospice)

  - 50% of these are admitted to a nursing home for rehabilitation or long-term care

- The total cost of hospital readmissions with a direct relationship to long-term care facilities was $4.34 billion (Mor et al., 2010)

Less obvious costs of rehospitalizations

Less obvious costs of rehospitalizations associated with LTCF residents are:

- Medical and nursing errors resulting in negative outcomes

- Numerous medication changes, each with the potential of adverse consequences

- Confusion, delirium, relocation trauma

- Stress, distress, and anxiety for residents, family members, and caregivers

- Complications such as falls, polypharmacy, adverse drug reactions, urinary tract infection, and pressure ulcers

- Duplication of tests or procedures

- Functional decline of residents

- Loss of revenue due to empty beds

Commitment

The Omnibus Budget Reconciliation Act of 1987 mandates that LTCFs ensure that residents attain or maintain their "highest practicable physical, mental, and psychosocial well-being." Facilities with a sincere desire to comply with the law have done an incredible job of using critical thinking, teamwork, learning their role and responsibilities, and developing and implementing creative and innovative programs. Having a formal program for preventing unnecessary readmissions to the hospital helps the residents attain or maintain their "highest practicable physical, mental, and psychosocial well-being."

Implementing new programs or changing existing practices requires a commitment from administration and nursing management, and a buy-in from staff. This is an investment of time, effort, and material resources with the potential for paying great dividends. Education is required to change practices, routines, and behaviors. Major change almost always affects the entire staff and all of the residents. Thorough planning and preparation will ensure the change is as smooth as possible. Teach by example. If mistakes are made, teach the proper response. Avoid a punitive approach. A successful program is achievable if you are inquisitive, a good teacher, a team player, and determined to make it work. Because there is no single evidence-based role model, use brainstorming and critical thinking to consider different methods that are realistic for your facility. Use the many tools at your disposal. Be determined and persistent. Success is definitely within your reach and, together with your team, you will make a difference in facility compliance, quality care, and quality of life for your residents!

Establishing or Modifying a Facilitywide Program

Calculate your rehospitalization rate and set a goal to reduce it by x% within the next year. To calculate this rate you must first determine the window of time when a readmission is considered a rehospitalization. For example, in your facility a hospital readmission occurs within 7, 15, or 30 days after the most recent hospital discharge. Medicare uses a seven-day benchmark for calculating readmission rates, but some facilities use a longer period of time.

- After you have identified your window time, count the number of residents who were readmitted to the hospital within the readmission window.

- Divide the number of residents who were readmitted by your average monthly census. For example, 10 residents were readmitted to the hospital. Your average census was 100 for the 30-day period.

- Divide the average census by the window time. For example, divide the census of 100 by 7 for a seven-day window, or divide 100 by 30 when using a 30-day window.

Ending Hospital Readmissions: A Blueprint for SNFs

- Divide the 10 readmissions by the average census window time to determine the answer.

- The equation for the readmission rate is written as residents readmitted/total residents admitted.

Considerations

The factors to consider in establishing or revising any program are:

- Regulation

  - Determine the requirements, how the program fits into the regulations in your state and measures to ensure compliance

- Reimbursement

  - What are the costs?

  - What are the ongoing program support (fixed, routine) costs?

  - How will the program be funded (if it is reimbursed at all) and, if so, how?

  - Will the program generate additional revenue?

- Rewards

  - What are the rewards for residents?

  - What are the rewards for staff?

  - What are the rewards for the facility?

  - Will the facility's image benefit?

Steps to take

Consider that some professionals may be more receptive to reporting from a person of equal status. Nursing supervisors, the director of nursing, and the attending physician should expect to be involved with some transitions. For all staff, consider the need for the following preliminary steps:

- Designate a task force of team members including nurses and nursing assistants

  - Assess documentation

  - Develop pathways and protocols

  - Develop policies and procedures

  - Identify training needs

- Be sure all shifts are represented

- Involve the medical director and attending physicians

- Develop an organizational goal for quality improvement efforts that focuses on preventing unnecessary rehospitalizations

- Determine accountability for the program and designate a nurse to oversee it

- Identify the specific role and responsibilities of each person (or position) involved with transitions. Emphasize individual accountability and provide clear feedback. These things are essential for positive outcomes.

- Teach staff the specific skills they must perform

  - Using problem solving activities is an excellent tool for teaching nurses

  - Role play is a good tool for teaching nursing assistants

– Fast facts for creative teaching, role playing, and other subjects are available at *www.chcf.org/fastfacts*

– Emphasize the need for good handwashing (or using alcohol-based products) and standard precautions

  ▪ Keep good records

  ▪ Validate competence

  ▪ Asking staff to submit a list of questions and problems is often very helpful. Addressing their problems acknowledges the importance of unit staff and shows you sincerely want to find solutions. Perhaps you can brainstorm solutions, but in any event, you are keeping communication open.

• Be sure that staff knows the difference between universal and standard precautions (Table 7.1) and has a solid working knowledge of transmission-based precautions.

• Orient staff to their responsibilities.

• Require hourly rounding on all residents by all nursing staff.

• Develop a means of identifying high-risk conditions, such as with a sticker or colored wristband.

• Develop protocols for nursing staff before calling the physician or healthcare provider.

• Unless it is a life or death emergency, call the healthcare provider first rather than sending the resident to the emergency room.

• Identify the most useful/helpful information to provide when reporting to the physician or health care provider or transitioning to another facility.

| Table 7.1 | Brief Comparison of Universal and Standard Precautions |

Universal Precautions (UP)	Standard Precautions (SP)
Universal precautions apply to:	Gloves for all contact with body substances and tissues, whether blood is visible
• Blood	
• Other body fluids containing visible blood semen, vaginal secretions	Includes:
• Tissues	• Blood
• Fluids: cerebrospinal, synovial, pleural, peritoneal, pericardial, and amniotic fluids	• Body fluid
	• Secretions
	• Excretions
Universal precautions do not apply to:	• Mucous membranes
• Feces	• Nonintact skin
• Nasal secretions	• Breast milk
• Sputum	
• Sweat	
• Tears	
• Urine	
• Vomitus	
• Saliva	
• Breast milk	
Unless these substances contain visible blood	
No provision for changing gloves during care; change gloves after each patient	Change gloves immediately prior to contact with mucous membranes and nonintact skin
Apply to items and surfaces that may have contacted substances to which UP apply	Apply to items and surfaces that may have contacted substances to which SP apply
Environmental contamination not an issue	Notes to avoid environmental contamination with used gloves
Avoid recapping needles	Avoid recapping needles
Splashing not addressed	Masks, eyewear, gowns if splashing likely

- Place a high priority on safe transitions and inform staff they are everyone's responsibility.

- Promote critical thinking and use of evidence-based assessment tools and pathways.

- Practice preventive care. Identify risk factors and the potential for complications. Intervene early.

- Develop a format for giving report at the bedside. Encourage collaborative assessment and documentation.

- Allow nursing assistants to share tasks. Get them involved and show that you value their opinions.

- Empower residents and families, such as by using family teaching tools and return demonstrations.

- Teach staff to do a comprehensive assessment when a change in condition has been identified.

- Identify residents who are at high risk of an acute change in condition and rehospitalization using the minimum data set (MDS) and other tools.

  – You may wish to triage residents according to their stability. Write care and monitoring protocols for each level.

  – Educate caregiving staff related to the importance of risk assessment, identification of risk, and ability to identify acute change of condition.

  – Identify causes of acute change of condition and feasibility of managing the resident in the nursing facility.

  – Manage the acute change of condition.

 – Integrate unplanned hospital transfers into ongoing quality improvement processes.

 – PointRight Inc. provides a clinical and risk management tool that measures resident outcomes affecting quality of care. Their tools can be used for rehospitalization prediction. The RADAR tool consists of a series of descriptive scores and predictive scales that are derived directly from the MDS 3.0. The report details resident risk factors and characteristics related to each of the scales. It also validates corporate compliance efforts by supporting the allocation of resources based on resident conditions. For additional information, see *www.pointright.com.*

• Develop a monitoring protocol for high risk residents.

• Residents with the high-risk conditions noted in this chapter should be monitored by a registered nurse every shift, using established monitoring protocols.

• Provide a list of things to monitor on resident charts. Refer to the example in the Appendix of your book.

• Identify the causes of acute changes of condition and determine whether it is feasible to manage the residents in the facility.

• Consider using the SBAR system of reporting, which is recommended by a number of experts:

 – S = situation

 – B = background

 – A = assessment

 – R = recommendation

- Establish reporting protocols using SBAR. You will find additional useful information at *http://consultgerirn.org/resources.* Refer to Dimension 10.

- Establish protocols for reporting change in condition from LTCF staff to physicians and other healthcare providers, and other facilities.

- Establish policies in which a supervisory nurse must assess the resident before any unplanned transfers, with the exception of life threatening emergencies.

- Use elements of American Medical Directors Association guidelines for communicating change in condition.

- Devise a checklist of things that must be done and documents that should accompany residents upon transfer.

- Develop protocols, pathways, or care maps for managing acute changes of condition. Develop specific pathways for:

  - Acute change in mental status

  - Fever

  - Dehydration

  - Electrolyte imbalance

  - Urinary tract infection

  - Pneumonia, lower respiratory tract infection

  - Sepsis

  - Congestive heart failure

  - Gastrointestinal distress

- Develop methods or templates for reporting symptoms of the above conditions.

- Educate family members and residents regarding the program.

- Determine a method of communication among and between departments, personnel, residents, families, and other community facilities, as appropriate.

  – Describe types of information to communicate at shift report

  – The off-going nurse should review resident status with oncoming nursing assistants

- Develop forms and other useful tools as needed.

  – Consider developing checklists, such as those for documenting resident education and pre- and post-transition activities, post discharge follow-ups, etc. (Chapter 8)

- Identify or develop tools that will help the facility meet program goals.

- Determine how and when the program will be integrated into facility's existing care and routines.

- Determine how monitoring will be done and who will do it.

- Determine the method of documentation to use, if this differs from your usual routine.

- Determine how to teach personnel, who to teach, how to motivate staff.

- Designate staff members who are responsible for arranging transitions, preparing transfer information, and answering questions before and after the transfer.

- Develop tracking systems and logs with beginning date and time and ending date and time.

- Establish a reward system. (See downloads page for more on employee incentives.)

- Complete the steps above before proceeding.

- Consider having therapy make a home visit for each person who is transitioning home.

The transitions program must:

- Have policies, procedures, measurable objectives, and interventions

- Show evidence of periodic assessment and evaluation

Philosophy of Care

Each facility should have an overall philosophy of care. This philosophy should incorporate efforts to monitor residents to provide quality care. If it does not, consider revising it or writing a simple philosophy statement to cover your program for preventing unnecessary rehospitalizations.

A philosophy is a statement of purpose. In this situation, the philosophy identifies your beliefs about the need for and provision of preventing unnecessary rehospitalizations.

- Determine your philosophy of care.

- Introduce a change in philosophy in the appropriateness of hospitalizations.

- Your actions should reflect both your words and philosophy. This is both talking the talk and walking the walk.

- The philosophy is a pledge or commitment to striving to ensure the residents will be assisted to attain and maintain their highest practicable level of functioning.

Director of Nursing

The director of nursing (DON) is responsible for overseeing nursing services and its programs and evaluating their effectiveness. He or she is responsible for making modifications or improvements to the overall program. The DON must be in tune with the program, promote the philosophy, and continuously evaluate the results. Create an environment of positive feedback and encouragement. The DON or designee should also ensure that:

- Staff understand the purpose, philosophy, and importance of this program.

- Ongoing continuing education is available to meet the needs of staff.

- Information about preventing unnecessary rehospitalizations is included in the nursing service orientation program.

- Monitoring tools are in place.

- Sufficient qualified staff is available to meet the needs of residents and ensure careful, accurate monitoring. Useful information on staffing is available at available at *http://consultgerirn.org/resources*. Refer to Dimension 12.

- The quality assurance committee reviews this program. As performance improvement needs develop, formulate action plans to ensure that the goals are met.

- Documentation reflects the provision of the nursing process, thorough monitoring, and quality care.

- Integrate unplanned hospitalizations into the quality improvement processes.

- Staff are familiar with state advance directive laws, when and how to use advance directives (Chapter 4.)

Consider appointing a transitions coordinator for your facility. This can be a part-time position in facilities with few admissions and discharges. Facilities that have many admissions and discharges each month will need a full-time person. The person in this position should work to build collaborative relationships with other facilities and healthcare providers in the area. This person should also ensure discharge teaching and followups are done. He or she should screen potential new admissions (and visit, if possible) before accepting the resident. The transitions coordinator should also work with family members to ensure quality, safety, and adherence to the resident's preferences. Recognize and accept nontraditional families, such as significant others and same sex partners. This is a cooperative program. Avoid placing 100% of the responsibility for the transition on a single staff person or family member. Your role is to teach, assist, and empower the involved individuals. If the resident is cognitively impaired, be sure the family caregiver has legal authority to act on the resident's behalf. You will find an example job description for this position in the Appendix of your book.

Managing Potential Barriers to Success

Consider systemic and individual resident barriers and how to manage or eliminate them. Consider ways of motivating residents and team members. Barriers can be a problem in any program, whether new or existing. Considering and identifying potential roadblocks and planning methods of eliminating them will benefit everyone.

Resident barriers

- Physical function

- Refusal of monitoring or care

- Lack of motivation

- Cognitive impairment, lack of cooperation

- Pain

- Fatigue

- Lack of knowledge or understanding

- Family/resident uncooperative

- Learned dependence

- Uses dependence as a means of getting attention, as a social contact, or exerting control over the environment (dependence is rewarded with attention; independence is not rewarded)

- Lack of rewards

Systemic barriers

- No assigned, qualified person to oversee the program or assigned person has too many responsibilities

- Lack of adequate staff

- Poor internal and external communication

- Lack of input from resident consumers and caregiving staff

- Facility emphasis on speed and efficiency

- Poor organization and time management skills

- Short staffing

- Uneducated or unqualified staff

- Lack of education, information, or preparation in preventing unnecessary rehospitalizations

- Unreasonable expectations of staff

- Poor communication

- Disorganization on the unit

- Staff with heavy resident assignments and/or inadequate time

- Excessive turnover at all levels

- Frequent turnover of nurse managers and/or director of nursing

- Lack of staff education or understanding

- Failure to completely and accurately assess the residents and identify their needs

- Care plan not used or not accessible

- Lack of understanding of reimbursement mechanisms

- Lack of understanding of MDS

- Inadequate system for completing and monitoring documentation of care

- Inadequate system for monitoring effectiveness of care

- Lack of managerial support

- Residents and unit staff are not aware of the program and its goals: everyone must be familiar with and buy into it

Nursing assistant barriers

- Many of the barriers above also apply to nursing assistants and are not duplicated here

- Inadequate supervision

- Nursing assistants not encouraged to use care plan

- Lack of support by nurses

- Heavy or unrealistic workload, inadequate staffing, and/or insufficient time

- No voice regarding policies, procedures, operations, things that affect nursing assistant practice

- Lack of information from nursing management

- Negative, calloused, and/or uncaring attitude

- Lack of confidence in self

- Lack of confidence in resident(s)

- Lack of belief in the philosophy or care

- Lack of an overall facility reward system

Obtain data

- Monthly readmission numbers

- Monthly emergency department transfers

- Determine potential drivers of readmissions

- Calculate the facility's current rate of rehospitalizations

- Analyze care delivery for strengths and weaknesses; address weaknesses

- Develop a plan to reduce unnecessary rehospitalizations

- Evaluate and prioritize improvement opportunities

- Monitor progress

- Work with community hospitals and other agencies

- Establish an effective means of communication to and from the facility

- Consider meeting with other agencies to develop a universal transfer form

- Improve documentation

- Enhance communication

- Aid in the early identification of a resident's change of condition

- Stabilize staff and increase hiring to improve the per patient day ratio so adequate monitoring can be done

- Take measures to reduce turnover

- Teach staff to manage residents with mental and behavioral health issues since many of the rehospitalizations occur with these residents

- Ensure that sufficient medical support is available, especially during late nights and weekends

Interact II

The Interact II program has a number of resources and excellent tools, pocket cards, and reporting guidelines for front line personnel to use in improving care and reducing avoidable hospital admissions. Several of these tools are appropriate for use by nursing assistants and other staff who have resident contact. This is an excellent resource for LTCFs. Refer to *http://interact.geriu.org/*

CHAPTER 8

Essential Elements of Smooth Transitions

Transition Initiatives

A number of initiatives are underway to reduce the incidence of rehospitalization. At the time of this writing, the most successful initiatives have common components. Consider implementing these approaches when making discharge preparations. These include:

- Appointing a staff member (usually a nurse) to plan and coordinate discharges and transitions to other settings. (Refer to the job description in the Chapter 7 Appendix.)

- Initiating discharge planning early.

- Identifying risk of readmission by using a validated tool or established criteria.

- Keeping the lines of communication open.

- Following up with the person by phone after discharge. The best results are achieved with longer and consistent follow-up

- Maintaining awareness of the person's condition during the postdischarge monitoring period and promptly intervening whenever necessary.

- Monitoring facility performance and results.

     – Keeping these data can be time consuming and expensive, but recordkeeping will help you to evaluate your transition procedures and make improvements in your program. Most facilities document, trend, and track pre- and post-discharge information records electronically.

Information on numerous related transition initiatives and programs is available at *www.ahrq.gov/qual/nhsurvey10/nhimpdim.htm.*

The Transition Survival Skills tool for residents and families is available at *www.caretransitions.org/transitionskills.asp.*

Resident-Centered Transitions

Care transitions should be resident-centered and always consider the resident's cultural health beliefs, preferences, literacy level, practices, and preferred language. Safe and effective resident-centered transitions involve conforming the transition to the resident, rather than asking the resident to accommodate the facility's needs. At one time, all records and paperwork stayed in the facility. In today's environment, certain documents stay with the resident. Excellent communication with the resident, family, and other healthcare providers is essential.

Readiness for Discharge

Prepare residents and their families for transitions whenever possible. Older adults typically have different discharge needs than those in younger age groups due to presence of multiple comorbidities, limitations related to illness, impaired mobility, reduced joint motion, anxiety, fatigue, cognitive impairment and other sensory impairments such as vision and hearing impairments, weakness and lack of stamina, health literacy deficits, and living alone. Discharge preparations may take much longer than expected.

Facilities should always weigh the benefits and risks before making a decision to transfer a resident. In addition to the risk of relocation trauma, consider the resident's wishes and other potential for harm. Make a decision to transfer the resident based on a match between the new setting and the resident's medical, nursing, and funct-ional needs. You may wish to refer to the American Medical Director's Association's (AMDA) "Acute Change of Condition in the Long-Term Care Settings." Transitions in which the long-term care facility (LTCF) may be involved include transitions from the:

- Facility to the acute care hospital

- Skilled nursing facility (SNF, Medicare level of care) to the nursing facility (NF, regular level of care)

- LTCF to an assisted living facility

- LTCF to the resident's own home or a relative's home with home health-care services

- LTCF to the resident's own home or a relative's home with a family or other caregiver

Nursing action

Your goal is to ensure the transition is as seamless and problem free as possible. If you have not familiarized yourself with the Interact II Toolkit, take a few minutes to do so. This is an invaluable tool with forms and other documents that will make the transi-tion much easier. Refer to *http://interact.geriu.org*.

Using a discharge readiness assessment is very helpful. Most of these were designed for acute care hospitals. A useful discharge preparation checklist that is appropriate for LTCF resident use is available at *www.caretransitions.org/documents/checklist.pdf.* Asking the resident or responsible party to complete this simple tool will help you identify areas in which teaching and resources are needed. A checklist that you can use to ensure you have met all your responsibilities may be downloaded from *http://tinyurl.com/2dygnz6.*

Risk for Readmission or Rehospitalization

Consider whether the resident is at risk for readmission or rehospitalization, such as residents with pending test results and those with fragile conditions. Those with multiple chronic medical problems are also at higher risk. Anticipate the need and develop a plan to reduce the risk, including delaying the transition until the resident's problems have been resolved. Other processes believed to be effective for ensuring smooth transitions and reducing the risk of readmission are:

- Risk screening

- Involving the resident's family

- Setting realistic goals and expectations in conjunction with the resident and family

- Coaching and care transition management

Communication

Clear communication is the foundation of resident safety and is essential to smooth transitions. Communication may be written or verbal, but both methods must be objective, concise, and complete. Fax and e-mail communication may also be used to communicate with the former resident and other parties involved in his or her care.

There is a great deal of confusion about the Health Insurance Portability and Account-ability Act's (HIPAA) release of information requirements that are applicable to transfers. Refer to Table 8.1 for information that should always accompany the resident or be sent to the receiving facility electronically. Likewise, your facility should expect to receive similar or comparable information from other facilities upon admission or readmission. In some states, you are expected to obtain documents such as the history and physical or discharge summary for incoming residents within a specified period of time. You may also be required to provide copies of these documents to the receiving organization at discharge. Table 8.2 lists myths and facts about the HIPAA privacy rule.

Pretransition Issues

Some activities that should be considered and completed before a nonemergency or scheduled transfer are listed here.

- If the facility does not have a transitions coordinator, specify one or more staff members to be responsible for a seamless transition.

- Discuss the transition with the resident and/or family as far in advance as feasible.

- Identify where the resident will go after discharge.

  - If the person will be discharging to a private residence, consider and plan for safety. Review the home safety information in the Appendix of your book and make preparations before the discharge date.

- Determine whether a caregiver is readily available when and where needed.

- Identify who will be providing the care and whether this level of care is likely to be adequate.

- In all probability, you will hand off care to this person.

Table 8.1	**Information to Accompany the Resident on Transfer to or From Another Facility**

Complete name
Primary diagnosis
Complete medication list or copy of facility medication record; note times of last doses and all recent as needed medications
Current vital signs; note if different from usual
Allergies
Advance directive
Code status
Facility phone and contact name
Family member or responsible party phone
Name of physician/primary care provider and contact information
Reason for transfer, including description of acute conditions and differences from resident's usual
Cognitive impairment, decision-making ability, health literacy
Medical devices and implants (e.g., insulin pump, dialysis, intrathecal pump, pacemaker, defibrillator, central line)
Recent test results
Test results pending
Tests that have been ordered but not completed
Diet order and ability to feed self/assistance needed
Level of independence with activities of daily living; note special help needed
Communication problems/special needs/language spoken (describe)
Vision (note use of glasses, contact lenses, presence of implants)
Hearing (note use of hearing aids, cochlear implant)
Dentures
Goals of care
Prognosis
If transferring to another long-term care facility, send MDS care plan, discharge plan, other documents required by state
If transferring home, send discharge plan, medication list, essential contact numbers, appointments, signs of danger and whom to call, other required documents

Table 8.2	HIPAA Myths and Facts

Myth	Fact
Receiving facilities cannot be provided with comprehensive resident information.	The Privacy Rule is balanced so that it permits the disclosure of personal health information needed for resident care and other important purposes. Releasing complete information is essential to smooth transitions and resident safety.
The Privacy Rule requires you to obtain a signed consent form before sharing information for treatment purposes.	The Privacy Rule *does not* require you to obtain a signed consent form before sharing information for treatment purposes. Healthcare providers can freely share information for treatment purposes without a signed authorization.
The Privacy Rule greatly limits all communications between you and the families and friends of residents.	The Privacy Rule does not cut off all communications between you and the families and friends of residents as long as the resident does not object to the information release. You are permitted to disclose information when needed to notify a family member or anyone responsible for the resident's care about the resident's location or general condition. You may share the appropriate information for these purposes even when the resident is incapacitated if doing so is in the best interest of the resident or required by law.
The Privacy Rule restricts calls and visits by family, friends, clergy, or anyone else.	Unless the resident objects, basic information such as phone number, room number, and general condition can be listed in the facility directory; be given to people who call or visit and ask for the resident; be given to clergy along with religious affiliation—when provided by the resident—even if the resident is not asked for by name.
The Privacy Rule is antielectronic.	The Privacy Rule *is not* antielectronic. You may communicate with residents, providers, and others by e-mail, telephone, or facsimile, with the implementation of appropriate safeguards to protect resident privacy.
Facilities may not communicate resident information by e-mail or fax.	The Privacy Rule does not prohibit the transfer of information electronically if appropriate safeguards are used.
Modified from: *www.hhs.gov/ocr/privacy/hipaa/understanding/coveredentities/cefastfacts.html.*	

Ending Hospital Readmissions: A Blueprint for SNFs

- Be sure this person is willing to assume responsibility for the resident.

- Experts suggest that you evaluate the identified caregiver for potential problems, needs, resources, and strengths and teaching needs related to the caregiving responsibility. The assessment is done from the caregiver's perspective and culture, and focuses on what assistance the caregiver may need and the outcomes the family member wants for support. The assessment also seeks to maintain the caregiver's own health and well-being. You may download assessment guidelines from *www.nextstepincare.org/uploads/File/ Assessing_Family_Caregivers2.pdf*.

  - Include caregiver needs and education in your teaching plan

- Try to anticipate and identify the resident's needs after discharge:

  - Include family caregivers as full partners in planning discharge and identifying home care needs

- These free publications may be useful:

  - Your Discharge Planning Checklist: For patients and their caregivers preparing to leave a hospital, nursing home, or other healthcare setting. Available at *www.medicare.gov/publications/pubs/pdf/11376.pdf*

  - Planning for Your Discharge: A checklist for patients and caregivers preparing to leave a hospital, nursing home, or other healthcare setting. Available at *www.caregiving.org/data/CMS_Discharge_Planning.pdf*

  - Care for the Family Caregiver: A Place to Start. Available at *www.caregiving.org/data/Emblem_CfC10_Final2.pdf*

  - Taking Charge of Your Healthcare: Your Path to Being an Empowered Patient. Available at *http://tinyurl.com/28brp59*

- Health Care Leader Action Guide to Reduce Avoidable Readmissions. Available at *www.hasc.org/download.cfm?ID=30374*

- Identify potential discharge barriers and make plans to minimize or eliminate them.

- Evaluate the care capacity of the home environment by discussing this with the resident, family members, therapists, and others who have made home visits.

- Use standard transfer and discharge-readiness criteria for residents with high-risk medical conditions.

Risks Associated With Poorly Executed Transitions

Thorough planning should precede each nonemergency transition. Poorly executed care transitions are dangerous for elderly persons. Transitions that are poorly planned and executed:

- Increase healthcare costs

- Are overly stressful for caregivers, families, and residents

- Compromise safety

- Lead to readmissions

Fragmented transitions can occur with any of the setting changes listed here. There is no single strategy or approach for managing transitions. Try to avoid fragmented transitions that have little communication and are accompanied by minimal information. This almost always results in a breakdown of care. One of the greatest problems is related to medication changes and dosage changes by personnel who are not familiar with the resident's history.

Predictors of poor postdischarge outcomes

Predictors of poor discharge outcomes include:

- Over age 80

- Multiple, active medical problems

- High-risk or unstable conditions, medical problems

- More than one hospitalization in the last six months

- Hospitalized within last 30 days

- Longer stay than expected or usual for condition

- History of depression

- Moderate to severe functional impairment

- Inadequate or unavailable support system

- Insecure, lacks self confidence to do self-care

- Failed discharge teaching (feedback, teachback)

- "Fair" or "poor" self-rating of health

- Poor, disabled, or on dialysis

- History of noncompliance with care or medications

High readmission rates have also been attributed to:

- Poor discharge transition coordination

- Inadequate teaching and discharge preparation

- Lack of resident and family caregiver readiness

- Difficulty coping with the demands of daily living

Postdischarge failures that increase the risk for rehospitalization

During the planning and teaching phase of the transition, consider all the problems and potential loopholes that increase the risk of failure. Develop a plan to reduce the risk. Common postdischarge failures include:

- Medication errors

- Discharge instructions that are confusing, contradictory to other instructions, need clarification, or not appropriate for the person's level of health literacy

- Lack of scheduled follow-up appointment with appropriate healthcare professionals, including specialists

- Appointments for follow-up physician visits not made soon enough

- Follow-up visit to the physician fell through because it was the sole responsibility of the client to secure a physician, make an appointment, and transfer records

- Inability of client to keep follow-up appointments because of illness or transportation problems

- Lack of an emergency plan with a number the person should call first

- Multiple healthcare providers are involved in the transition, resulting in client confusion about which provider is in charge

- Lack of strong social support

- Client lack of adherence to self-care activities (e.g., medications, therapies, daily weighing, wound care) because of confusion about needed care, availability of transportation, method for scheduling appointments, or how to access or pay for medications

Teaching

- Identify areas in which resident and/or family education are needed:

  - Synthesize the information and use it to prepare and implement a teaching plan.

  - Identify and include all parties who need to know this information in your teaching plan.

  - It may be necessary for the physical or occupational therapist to assist with some things, such as safety teaching and evaluating the home for accessibility and use of adaptive devices.

  - Residents are partners in their care and safety is enhanced by teaching residents and their families about their responsibilities in facilitating safe care. Explain that they are responsible for reporting perceived risk, and for asking questions if they do not understand procedures.

  - Start teaching well in advance so the resident has time to master the information or activity.

- Document all teaching activities

- Obtain feedback to ensure teaching was effective and understood:

  - The practice of asking residents to restate what they have learned in their own words is one of the 11 top resident safety practices (AHRQ, 2010).

  - If you identify a lack of understanding, provide additional teaching followed by another request for feedback.

- Ensure the resident and family are familiar with signs, symptoms, and potential problems, as well as when to call for help:

  – Prepare a postdischarge plan of care in conjunction with the resident and family that includes:

    ▪ The resident's continuing care needs

    ▪ The resident's and family's preferences for care

    ▪ Social and cultural preferences and issues

    ▪ How the needs will be met

    ▪ How the resident and family will access needed services

    ▪ How care should be coordinated if continuing treatment involves multiple caregivers

    ▪ Physical needs after discharge such as personal care, sterile dressings, and physical therapy

    ▪ A description of resident/caregiver education needs and how to best meet care needs after discharge

- Use this plan for discharge teaching activities

- Provide the discharge plan information in written format to the resident at the time of discharge and forward it to other authorized persons and agencies, with the consent of the resident or legal representative

Preparing Paperwork

- Follow facility policies for preparing medical information for the transition.

- Develop forms and templates to use to simplify the process.

- Designate a person to copy and assemble medical information for the transfer.

- Keep written discharge instructions as simple as possible. Be sure they are appropriate for the person's culture, health literacy, and current health status.

- Review the information you will be sending home to sure it is not too complicated, confusing, contradictory to other instructions, or inappropriate for the client's situation. It should be simple, legible, and easily understood. During discharge teaching sessions, ask clarifying questions about the instructions and plan of care to ensure the information was understood.

- Provide the resident's primary care provider with relevant discharge and medical information in one packet rather than one document at a time.

Advance Directives

Review advance directives with the resident and/or responsible party to ensure they reflect the resident's current wishes. Provide documents for the resident to update, if needed. If the resident does not have a directive, offer the opportunity to complete one at this time.

Check your state's website to see if special forms, such as out-of-hospital directives, are available. Some states also have forms for unmarried domestic partners and forms to use when a person has not executed or issued a directive and is incompetent or incapable of communication. These forms change frequently, so check the website regularly. Websites with multi-state information on advance directives are:

- *http://hippo.findlaw.com/hippoadv.html*

- *http://tinyurl.com/23kturw*

- *www.familydecisions.org*

Medications

- Provide medication teaching and answer medication-related questions

  - Explain that the resident should take only listed medications and avoid drugs used previously that are not listed

  - Stress the need for accuracy of the medication regimen

- Complete the medication reconciliation process

  - Consider having the facility pharmacist review the final medication list

  - If you are not familiar with medication reconciliation, you may wish to download Getting Started Kit: Prevent Adverse Drug Events (Medication Reconciliation) How-to Guide from *http://tinyurl.com/24469ge*

  - The medication reconciliation and discrepancy tools in the Appendix of your book are also useful for facilitating reconciliation of medication across settings and prescribers

- After all parties have reviewed the reconciled medications, provide the resident with a complete and accurate list that includes drug names, dosage, frequency, reason, special monitoring, and potential side effects

- Inquire about the resident's ability to acquire medications; also consider cost and transportation to the pharmacy:

    – Discuss the need for calling for refills 24 to 72 hours in advance

    – If the resident has orders for schedule II drugs, he or she should be aware that prescriptions may need to be picked up in person

Other Preparatory Activities

Make arrangements for:

    – Durable medical equipment (e.g., oxygen, hospital bed, commode, trapeze)

    – Necessary medical supplies

    – Physician appointments

    – Other appointments, including those for diagnostic tests

    – Support services (e.g., home healthcare, meal service programs)

    – Prepare and provide a list of community resources such as home healthcare and community meal service programs

- Assist the resident to prepare and maintain a personal record that he or she brings to all appointments and keeps current at all times. An example form is in the Appendix of your book.

- Secure transportation for the transition, if needed

Coordination With Others

Contact all parties who will be providing care and services for the resident after discharge, including the following:

- Stay in contact with the primary care physician or healthcare provider to ensure he or she is involved with discharge planning.

- Notify the attending physician at the time of discharge so he or she is aware that the person has returned to a lesser care setting or independent living situation in the community.

- If a different physician is assuming responsibility for the client's care in the community, contact the physician and provide background information. Fax or mail information as needed. Provide a contact name at the facility in case additional information is needed.

- Ensure that follow-up appointments are made.

- Coordinate services among sequential providers.

    - If the resident is going to a lower level of care, contact the receiving facility or agency to orient staff and communicate the resident's individual needs

    - If the resident is to be discharged to a lower level of care (e.g., board and care home, assisted living facility, home healthcare services), provide transfer information (estimated time of arrival, transportation, etc.) and assess whether the organization's personnel are engaged and ready to participate in care as needed

    - Confirm the receiving facility's (or agency's) readiness to receive the resident

Home Discharges

When residents are discharging to a home setting:

- Give the family a list of safety factors in the home. Ask them to make preparations to reduce the risk of accidents. (See the Appendix of your book.)

- Provide a medication reconciliation list.

- Be sure the resident and family caregiver know what each medication is, when to take it, and where to get it.

- Teach the resident and family caregiver signs of complications or danger and who to call if they occur.

- Confirm the resident and family caregiver's ability to attend follow up appointments.

- Verify that the resident and family caregiver understand any activity limitations and can follow a special diet, if ordered.

- If the resident will be living alone or with a spouse, consider the need for other community services.

- Prepare and provide a list of community resources such as home healthcare, transportation, and meal delivery programs.

Other Miscellaneous Issues

- Work with the resident's family to gather and return possessions, ensuring nothing is lost. As possessions are removed, have the resident's personal inventory signed.

- Document the steps and preparations for transition or keep a checklist.

- Identify the next steps in the resident's care and assist in making referrals, as needed.

- Provide support to the resident and family as needed.

- Forward all information to other persons and agencies promptly.

Steps to Take Immediately Before Discharge

- Immediately before discharge, assess the resident to ensure he or she is stable for transfer

  - Numerous useful geriatric assessment tools are available at *http://consultgerirn.org/resources*. Refer to Dimension 9.

At the time of discharge, confirm that the resident and family caregiver:

- Know what medication to take and where to get it

- Know the signs and symptoms of danger and who to call if they occur

- Have made a prompt follow-up appointment with the community physician and are able to keep it

  - Have arranged for transportation to appointments, if needed

- Understand and can verbalize the resident's diet and activity limitations

Postdischarge Activities

Complete the discharge summary that includes:

- A recapitulation of the resident's stay

- A final summary of the resident's status

Ending Hospital Readmissions: A Blueprint for SNFs

Complete the discharge information on the minimum data set. At one time, facilities gave little thought to residents who were discharged. This is no longer the case. Your postdischarge responsibilities are essential to a seamless and safe transition. Your goals for discharge and beyond are to prevent errors, ensure safety, and prevent rehospitalizations. A bonus is that following the resident for a period of time after discharge enhances confidence, builds good will and positive regard, and augments satisfaction for the client and family. Avoid making promises that you cannot keep during phone contact with the client.

Postdischarge monitoring

Facility discharge is a stressful time. Residents should sign the acknowledgment you provide for discharge teaching. However, despite being given a copy of the discharge instructions, many never look at the paperwork again. Residents and families may feel overwhelmed with the amount of paper and instructions for which they are accountable at the time of discharge. If this is the case, they have difficulty coping and some will turn to the emergency room for help and end up being rehospitalized. Give the client and family business cards with the name and phone number for the facility contact person (transitions coordinator). Inform them that someone will be calling to check on them periodically. Invite them to call the facility contact if they have questions or problems. If the transition coordinator is not available, invite them to call the discharging unit. Facilities who have studied call backs have found that most calls fall into these categories:

- Asking questions and seeking medication clarification, 83%

- Problems that were subsequently redirected to the physician or other care provider, 8%

- Problems that were subsequently referred to the emergency room, 9%

Residents who were recently discharged may experience complications that lead to the need for readmission to either the LTCF, the acute care hospital, or both. Telephone the former resident 24 to 48 hours after discharge to check on the person's well-being. Speak with both the client (former resident; now technically a client) and family caregiver, if possible. Calling a client and/or family members shows that the facility sincerely cares about the person and his or her safety and takes the responsibility for transitions seriously.

When speaking with the client and caregiver:

- Ask the client and caregiver if they have problems, needs, issues, or questions that you can assist with.

- Ask the client how they are feeling. Do they need assistance scheduling a physician appointment?

- Ensure that the client has necessary medical supplies, medications, and equipment.

- Remind the client of follow-up appointments, importance of seeing the physician, etc.

- Follow up with the client on specific events such as doctor appointments or home healthcare visits.

- Ask about the client's progress toward their stated goal since the last contact. Provide positive reinforcement.

- Determine whether expected community resources have been initiated.

- Ask about home health visits.

- Discuss medications and treatments to ensure there are no problems.

  - Medication errors are a problem in all settings, so determine if the person is taking his or her medications correctly

Ending Hospital Readmissions: A Blueprint for SNFs

- Identify the need for additional resources not previously anticipated.

- Ask questions about the condition for which the client was in the LTCF:

  – Ask about symptoms of chronic disease (e.g., congestive heart failure), if applicable

  – If the client was in the LTCF for therapy or another service, ask about physical function, weight bearing, weakness, level of independence or need for assistance with activities of daily living, etc.

  – If the client was treated for infection, ask about signs and symptoms

  – Inquire about red flags and specific problems

- It may also be necessary to assist with:

  – Prioritizing and organizing daily self-care

  – Help the person with self-management skills and resources, as needed

  – Providing assistance in learning self-care or making a referral to a community resource

- Make referrals to other services, if indicated.

References

1. Alspaach, JoAnn Grif. 2010. "Weekend Admissions to Critical Care: Why Do More of These Patients Die?" *Critical Care Nurse* 30:10–12.

2. Aujesky, Drahomir, David Jiménez, Maria K. Mor, et al. 2009. "Weekend Versus Weekday Admission and Mortality After Acute Pulmonary Embolism." *Circulation* 119:962–8.

3. Bell, Chaim M., and Donald A. Redelmeier. 2001. "Mortality Among Patients Admitted to Hospitals on Weekends as Compared with Weekdays." *New England Journal of Medicine* 345:663–8.

4. Bobay, Kathleen L., Teresa A. Jerofke, Marianne Weiss, et al. 2010. "Age-Related Differences in Perception of Quality of Discharge Teaching and Readiness for Hospital Discharge." *Geriatric Nursing* 31(3):178–87.

5. Bohan, J. Stephen. 2007. "MI Mortality Worse for Weekend Admissions: Availability of Invasive Procedures Might be the Cause of Differential Mortality." *Journal Watch Emergency Medicine* March 16.

6. Boockvar, Kenneth S., Ann L. Gruber-Baldini, Lynda Burton, et al. 2005. "Outcomes of Infection in Nursing Home Residents With and Without Early Hospital Transfer." *Journal of the American Geriatrics Society* 53:590–6.

7. Boutwell, Amy, F. Griffin, S. Hwu S, et al. 2009. *Effective Interventions to Reduce Rehospitalizations: A Compendium of 15 Promising Interventions*. Cambridge, MA: Institute for Healthcare Improvement.

8. Caranasos, George J. 2002. "Drug Effects in the Elderly in Health Management of Older Adults II." Accessed September 30. *http://medinfo.ufl.edu/cme/hmoa2/*.

9. Cavallazzi, Rodrigo, Paul E. Marik, Amyn Hirani, et al. 2010. "Association Between Time of Admission to the ICU and Mortality: A Systematic Review and Metaanalysis." *Chest* 138(1): 68–75.

10. Centers for Medicare and Medicaid Services. 2010. *State Operations Manual.* Appendix PP - Guidance to Surveyors for Long Term Care Facilities (Rev 66, 10-01-10). Baltimore, MD: Author.

11. Centers for Medicare and Medicaid Services. 2010. *State Operations Manual.* Appendix A - Survey Protocol, Regulations and Interpretive Guidelines for Hospitals (Rev. 47, 06-05-09). Baltimore, MD: Author.

12. Coleman, Eric A., Carla Parry, Sandra Chalmers, et al. 2006. "The Care Transitions Intervention: Results of a Randomized Controlled Trial." *Archives of Internal Medicine* 166(17):1822–8.

13. Coleman, Eric A., Jodi D. Smith, Devbani Raha, et al. 2005. "Post-Hospital Medication Discrepancies: Prevalence, Types and Contributing Factors." *Archives of Internal Medicine* 165(16):1842–7.

14. Dosa, David. 2005. "Should I Hospitalize My Resident with Nursing Home-Acquired Pneumonia?" *Journal of the American Medical Directors Association* 6:327–33.

15. Ensminger, S. Allen, Ian J. Morales, Steve G. Peters, et al. 2004. "The Hospital Mortality of Patients Admitted to the ICU on Weekends." *Chest* 126:1292–8.

16. Foss, N. B., and H. Kehlet. 2006. "Short-term Mortality in Hip Fracture Patients Admitted During Weekends and Holidays." *British Journal of Anaesthesiology* 96(4):450–4.

17. Fried, T., M. Gillick, and L. Lipsitz. 1997. "Short-term Functional Outcomes of Long-term Care Residents with Pneumonia Treated with and without Hospital Transfer." *Journal of the American Geriatrics Society* 45:302–306.

18. Jack, Brian W., Veerappa K. Chetty, David Anthony, et al. 2009. "A Reengineered Hospital Discharge Program to Decrease Rehospitalization: A Randomized Trial." *Annals of Internal Medicine* 150(3):178–87.

19. James, Matthew T., Ron Wald, and Chaim M. Bell, et al. 2010. "Weekend Hospital Admission, Acute Kidney Injury, and Mortality." *Journal of the American Society of Nephrology* 21:728–31.

20. Kayser-Jones, Jeanie, Joyce Chan, and Alison Kris. 2004. "A Model Long-Term Care Hospice Unit: Care, Community, and Compassion." *Geriatric Nursing* 26(1):16–20.

21. Kind, Amy J, Maureen A. Smith, Nancy Pandhi, et al. 2007. "Bouncing-Back: Patterns and Predictors of Complicated Transitions Thirty Days after Hospitalization for Acute Ischemic Stroke." *Journal of the American Geriatric Society* 55(3):365–73.

22. Kruse, Robin L., David R. Mehr, Keith E. Boles, et al. 2004. "Does Hospitalization Impact Survival After Lower Respiratory Infection in Nursing Home Residents? *Medical Care* 42:860–70.

23. Kuijsten, Hans A., Sylvia Brinkman, Iwan A. Meynaar, et al. 2010. "Hospital Mortality is Associated with ICU Admission Time." *Intensive Care Medicine* 36:1765–71.

24. Leland, John. 2010. "A Battle Against Prescription Drugs Causes Pain." *New York Times*. Accessed October 2. *http://www.nytimes.com/2010/10/03/us/03rules.html*.

25. Loeb, Mark, Soo Chan Carusone, Ron Goeree, et al. 2006. "Effect of a Clinical Pathway to Reduce Hospitalizations in Nursing Home Residents with Pneumonia: A Randomized Controlled Trial." *Journal of the American Medical Association* 295:2503–10.

26. McCook, Alison. 2010. "Weekend Strokes More Deadly—But Why?" *Reuters Health*. Accessed on November 3. *http://www.reuters.com/article/idUSTRE6A04Z420101101*.

Ending Hospital Readmissions: A Blueprint for SNFs

27. Miller, Susan C., Julie C. Lima, and Susan L. Mitchell. 2010. "Hospice Care Increasing for Nursing Home Patients with Dementia." Accessed December 11. *http://aja.sagepub.com/content/25/8/666.abstract.*

28. Mor, Vincent, Orna Intrator, Zhanlian Feng, et al. 2010. "The Revolving Door of Rehospitalization From Skilled Nursing Facilities." *Health Affairs* 29(1):57–64.

29. Naylor, Mary, Dorothy Brooten, Robert Jones, et al. 1994. "Comprehensive Discharge Planning for the Hospitalized Elderly. A Randomized Clinical Trial." *Annals of Internal Medicine* 120(12):999–1006.

30. Naylor, Mary, Dorothy Brooten, Roberta Campbell, et al. 1999. "Comprehensive Discharge Planning and Home Follow-up of Hospitalized Elders: A Randomized Clinical Trial." *Journal of the American Medical Association* 281(7):613–20.

31. Naylor, Mary, Dorothy Brooten, Roberta Campbell, et al. 2004. "Transitional Care of Older Adults Hospitalized with Heart Failure: A Randomized, Controlled Trial." *Journal of the American Geriatric Society* 52(5):675–84.

32. Peberdy, Mary Ann, Joseph P. Ornato, G. Luke Larkin, et al. 2008. "Survival From In-hospital Cardiac Arrest During Nights and Weekends." *Journal of the American Medical Association* 299(7):785–92.

33. Ryan, Katheryn, Katharine Levit, and P. Hannah Davis. 2010. "Characteristics of Weekday and Weekend Hospital Admissions." HCUP Statistical Brief #87. March 2010. Agency for Healthcare Research and Quality, Rockville, MD. Accessed December 3. *http://www.hcup-us.ahrq.gov/reports/statbriefs/sb87.pdf.*

34. Sager et al., 1996.

35. Sakhuja, Ankit. 2010. "Weekend Admissions May Raise Death Risk in Kidney Patients." Accessed December 17. *http://health.usnews.com/health-news/family-health/digestive-disorders/articles/2010/11/19/weekend-admissions-may-raise-death-risk-in-kidney-patients.html.*

36. Saposnik, G. 2007.

37. Senelick, Richard C. 2010. "The 'Bounce Back Effect': How Hospital Readmissions Are Jeopardizing Medicare." Accessed October 27. *http://www.huffingtonpost.com/richard-c-senelick-md/the-bounce-back-effect-ho_b_677575.html?view=print.*

38. Smith, Jodi D., Eric A. Coleman, and Sung-Joo Min. 2004. "Identifying Post-Acute Medication Discrepancies in Community Dwelling Older Adults: A New Tool." *American Journal of Geriatric Pharmacotherapy* 2(2):141–8.

Ending Hospital Readmissions: A Blueprint for SNFs

39. Tobias, Dianne E., and Mark Sey. 2001. "General and Psychotherapeutic Medication Use in 328 Nursing Facilities: A Year 2000 National Survey." *Consultant Pharmacist* 16(1):54–64.

40. van Walraven, Carl, and Chaim M. Bell. 2002. "Risk of Death or Readmission Among People Discharged From Hospital on Fridays." *Journal of the Canadian Medical Association* 166(13):1672–3.

CHAPTER 1

Appendix

Facility Definitions 153

Twenty Key Conditions 156

Hospital Discharge Planning Requirements 157

Hospitals With the Highest Readmission Rates, 2010 169

Hospitals With the Lowest Readmission Rates, 2010 170

Facility Definitions

F150

§483.5 Definitions

(a) Facility defined. For purposes of this subpart "facility" means, a skilled nursing facility (SNF) or a nursing facility (NF) which meets the requirements of §§1819 or 1919(a), (b), (c), and (d) of the Social Security Act, the Act. "Facility" may include a distinct part of an institution specified in §440.40 of this chapter, but does not include an institution for the mentally retarded or persons with related conditions described in §440.150 of this chapter. For Medicare and Medicaid purposes (including eligibility, coverage, certification, and payment), the "facility" is always the entity which participates in the program, whether that entity is comprised of all of, or a distinct part of a larger institution. For Medicare, a SNF (see §1819(a)(1)), and for Medicaid, a NF (see §1919(a)(1)) may not be an institution for mental diseases as defined in §435.1009.

Interpretive Guidelines §483.5

The following are the statutory definitions at §§1819(a) and 1919(a) of the Act for a SNF and a NF:

"Skilled nursing facility" is defined as an institution (or a distinct part of an institution) which is primarily engaged in providing skilled nursing care and related services for residents who require medical or nursing care, or rehabilitation services for the rehabilitation of injured, disabled, or sick persons, and is not primarily for the care and treatment of mental diseases; has in effect a transfer agreement (meeting the requirements of §1861(l)) with one or more hospitals having agreements in effect under §1866; and meets the requirements for a SNF described in subsections (b), (c), and (d) of this section.

"Nursing facility" is defined as an institution (or a distinct part of an institution) which is primarily engaged in providing skilled nursing care and related services for residents who require medical or nursing care, rehabilitation services for the rehabilitation of injured, disabled, or sick persons, or on a regular basis, health-related care and services to individuals who because of their mental or physical condition require care and services (above the level of room and board) which can be made available to them only through institutional facilities, and is not primarily for the care and treatment of mental diseases; has in effect a transfer agreement (meeting the requirements of §1861(l)) with one or more hospitals having agreements in effect under §1866; and meets the requirements for a NF described in subsections (b), (c), and (d) of this section.

If a provider does not meet one of these definitions, it cannot be certified for participation in the Medicare and/or Medicaid programs.

NOTE: If the survey team finds substandard care in §§483.13, 483.15, or 483.25, follow the instructions for partial extended or extended surveys.

Other Types of Long-Term Care Facilities	
Long-Term Acute Care Hospital (LTACH)	A rapidly growing segment of the hospital market. The facility is a licensed hospital but is designed for patients who are expected to have a lengthy stay. To be accepted, the patient must have a medically complex condition, need acute care services, and have a good chance of improvement. The level of care is higher than provided in long-term care facilities (nursing homes) or subacute care facilities.
Rehabilitation hospital	This type of facility is devoted to medical rehabilitation, not substance rehabilitation. A licensed hospital that provides intensive rehabilitation and restorative services to patients following disease, illness, or injury. People entering this facility are not sick enough to remain in the acute care hospital. They are medically stable, but still need a great deal of care. The services are designed to help the person learn to function at the highest level possible. The facility will teach the person ADL skills and work with family members to determine what will be needed when the patient is released. Stay in this type of facility is usually lengthy.
Subacute Care Facility	Some of these are freestanding, and others are separate units within a licensed hospital or skilled nursing facility. Patients are medically stable, but require frequent assessment and higher level skills than an SNF. The patient may transfer to a skilled nursing facility when treatment is completed.
Intermediate-Care Facility for the Mentally Retarded (ICF/MR)	A freestanding facility that provides care for individuals with mental retardation or developmental disabilities. Habilitation services are provided based on client needs and level of disability. Clients may live in these facilities for life. The goals of care are to assist clients to be as independent as possible and provide the highest quality of life possible. Staff help clients achieve their potential through education and training.
Home Health Care	Provide health care services in the person's home for those who are recovering from illness or injury, are disabled, or are chronically or terminally ill. Services may include skilled nursing care; assistance with activities of daily living, housekeeping; social services; physical, occupational, respiratory, and speech therapy; emergency response; nutrition counseling; and case management.
Continuing Care Retirement Community (CCRC); may be called a Life Care Facility	Offers many levels of accommodation, from independent living to skilled nursing care. Some have special units, such as those for care of persons with Alzheimer's disease. The philosophy is that residents can age in place and do not have to leave the community if their needs change.
Assisted Living Facility (ALF)	Assisted living is designed for persons who need some assistance with activities of daily living, but do not need routine medical or nursing care. Non-licensed staff are the primary caregivers. As a rule, no licensed professionals are on duty 24 hours a day. If regular nursing care is needed, a home health agency may come in to provide the service. Residents are encouraged to be as independent and autonomous as possible.
Hospice	Hospice care has evolved around the philosophy that death is a natural process that should neither be hastened nor delayed and that the dying person should be kept comfortable. Hospice care is given to persons who are terminally ill people with a life expectancy of six months or less. It may be provided in special hospice facilities, in other care facilities, and at home. A team of workers assist both the terminally ill person and his family. The goals of hospice care are: • Control of pain • Coordinating psychological, spiritual, and social support services for the patient and the family • Making legal and financial counseling available to the patient and family
Adult Day Care	Families who work or are unable to provide supervision for a family member due to job responsibilities or other obligations often use adult day care. The person returns home in the evening. Programs offer health screening and oversight, meals, social and recreational activities.

Ending Hospital Readmissions: A Blueprint for SNFs

Twenty Key Conditions

Key Diagnostic Groups		
Diagnosis	Incidence Rate	Share of Total Spending per 1000 beneficiaries with episodes
1 Ischemic heart disease	20	14.0%
2 CHF	8.0	4.3%
3 Hypertension	44.0	4.0%
4 Cerebral vascular accident	8.0	3.6%
5 COPD	7.0	3.4%
6 Diabetes	18.0	3.2%
7 Joint degeneration - knee and lower leg	7.0	3.1%
8 Joint degeneration - back	12.0	3.0%
9 Chronic renal failure	4.0	2.8%
10 Closed fracture or dislocation - thigh, hip & pelvis	1.0	2.3%
11 Cataract	24.0	2.3%
12 Bacterial lung infections	4.0	2.1%
13 Malignant neoplasm of pulmonary system	1.0	1.6%
14 Malignant neoplasm of prostate	3.0	1.4%
15 Malignant neoplasm of breast	3.0	1.4%
16 Psychotic & schizophrenic disorders	2.0	1.3%
17 Malignant neoplasm of skin, major	8.0	1.2%
18 Joint degeneration - thigh, hip and pelvis	2.0	1.2%
19 Other metabolic disorders	6.0	1.2%
20 Atherosclerosis	3.0	1.3%

Source: "Greatest total Medicare spending and fast growing episodes"; Podulka, J.; MedPac; September 18, 2009 meeting presentation accessed 2010 February 19

Hospital Discharge Planning Requirements

Plans of care and discharge plans should be initiated immediately upon admission and be modified as patient care needs change.

§482.13(b)(1) The patient has the right to participate in the development and implementation of his or her plan of care.

Interpretive Guidelines §482.13(b)(1)

This regulation requires the hospital to actively include the patient in the development, implementation, and revision of his or her plan of care. It requires the hospital to plan the patient's care, with patient participation, to meet the patient's psychological and medical needs.

The patient's (or patient's representatives, as allowed by state law) right to participate in the development and implementation of his or her plan of care includes, at a minimum, the right to participate in the development and implementation of his or her inpatient treatment/care plan or outpatient treatment/care plan, participate in the development and implementation of his or her discharge plan, and participate in the development and implementation of his or her pain management plan.

Informed decisions related to care planning also extend to discharge planning for the patient's postacute care. See the guidelines at 42 CFR 482.43(c) pertaining to discharge planning for discussion of pertinent requirements.

§482.43 Condition of Participation: Discharge Planning
The hospital must have in effect a discharge planning process that applies to all patients. The hospital's policies and procedures must be specified in writing.

Interpretive Guidelines §482.43

This Condition of Participation (CoP) applies to all types of hospitals and requires all hospitals to conduct appropriate discharge planning activities for all inpatients. It applies to patients who are admitted to the hospital as inpatients. This CoP does not apply to patients who appear in a hospital emergency department but are not admitted as hospital inpatients.

The written discharge planning process must reveal a thorough, clear, and comprehensive process that is understood by the hospital staff.

Adequate discharge planning is essential to the health and safety of all patients. Patients may suffer adverse health consequences upon discharge without benefit of appropriate planning. Such planning is vital to mapping a course of treatment aimed at minimizing the likelihood of having any patient rehospitalized for reasons that could have been prevented.

§482.43(a) Standard: Identification of Patients in Need of Discharge Planning
The hospital must identify at an early stage of hospitalization all patients who are likely to suffer adverse health consequences upon discharge if there is no adequate discharge planning.

Interpretive Guidelines §482.43(a)

Medicare participating hospitals are afforded great flexibility in setting the criteria for identifying patients who are likely to suffer adverse health consequences upon discharge without adequate discharge planning. Presently, there is no nationally accepted tool or criteria for identifying these individuals. However, the following factors have been identified as important: functional status, cognitive ability of the patient, and family support.

Patients at high risk for requiring posthospital services must be identified through a screening process. The hospital should reevaluate the needs of the patients on an ongoing basis and prior to discharge, as the needs may change based on the individual's status.

There is no set time frame for identification of patients requiring a discharge planning evaluation other than it must be done as early as possible. The timing is left up to the hospital, its staff, and attending MD/DO.

§482.43(b) Standard: Discharge Planning Evaluation
(1) The hospital must provide a discharge planning evaluation to the patients identified in paragraph (a) of this section, and to other patients upon the patient's request, the request of a person acting on the patient's behalf, or the request of the physician.

Interpretive Guidelines §482.43(b)(1)

The needs assessment can be formal or informal. A needs assessment generally includes an assessment of factors that impact a patient's needs for care after discharge from the acute care setting. These may include assessment of biopsychosocial needs, the patient's and caregiver's understanding of discharge needs, and identification of posthospital care resources.

At the present time, there is no nationally accepted standard for the evaluation. The purpose of a discharge planning evaluation is to determine continuing care needs after the patient leaves the hospital setting. It is not intended to be a care-planning document. The hospital may develop an evaluation tool or protocol.

§482.43(b)(2) - A registered nurse, social worker, or other appropriately qualified personnel must develop, or supervise the development of, the evaluation.

Interpretive Guidelines §482.43(b)(2)

The responsibility for discharge planning is often multidisciplinary. It is not restricted to a particular discipline. The hospital has flexibility in designating the responsibilities of the registered nurse, social worker, or other appropriate qualified personnel for discharge planning. The responsible personnel should have experience in discharge planning, knowledge of social and physical factors that affect functional status at discharge, and knowledge of community resources to meet postdischarge clinical and social needs.

Ideally, discharge planning will be an interdisciplinary process, involving disciplines with specific expertise, as dictated by the needs of the patient. For example, for a patient with emphysema, the discharge planner could coordinate respiratory therapy and nursing care, and financial coverage for home care services and oxygen equipment, and patient/caregiver education using cost-effective, available community services in an expedient manner.

§482.43(b)(3) - The discharge planning evaluation must include an evaluation of the likelihood of a patient needing posthospital services and of the availability of the services.

Interpretive Guidelines §482.43(b)(3)

The hospital is responsible for developing the discharge plan for patients who need a plan and for arranging its initial implementation. The hospital's ability to meet discharge planning requirements is based on the following:

- Implementation of a needs assessment process with identified high-risk criteria;

- Evidence of a complete, timely, and accurate assessment;

- Maintenance of a complete and accurate file on community-based services and facilities including long term care, sub acute care, home care or other appropriate levels of care to which patients can be referred; and

- Coordination of the discharge planning evaluation among various disciplines responsible for patient care.

§482.43(b)(4) - The discharge planning evaluation must include an evaluation of the likelihood of a patient's capacity for self-care or of the possibility of the patient being cared for in the environment from which he or she entered the hospital.

Interpretive Guidelines §482.43(b)(4)

The capacity for self-care includes the ability and willingness for such care. The choice of a continuing care provider depends on the self-care components, as well as availability, willingness, the ability of family/caregivers, and the availability of resources.

The hospital must inform the patient or family as to their freedom to choose among providers of posthospital care. Patient preferences should also be considered; however, preferences are not necessarily congruent with the capacity for self- care.

Patients should not only be evaluated for return to the prehospital environment, but also should be offered a range of realistic options to consider for posthospital care. This includes patients admitted to a hospital from a SNF, who should be evaluated to determine an appropriate discharge site. Hospital staff should incorporate information provided by the patient and/or caregivers to implement the process.

The Social Security Act (SSA) at §1861(ee) requires Medicare-participating hospitals, as part of their discharge planning evaluations, share with each patient, as appropriate, a list of Medicare-certified home health agencies (HHA) that serve the geographic area in which the patient resides and that request to be included on the list. In addition, the SSA prohibits hospitals from limiting or steering patients to any particular HHA and must identify those HHA to which the patient is referred in which the hospital has a disclosable financial interest or in which the HHA has an interest in the hospital.

The SSA, section 1861(ee) requires a hospital's discharge plan to include an evaluation of the patient's likely need for hospice care and posthospital extended care services and to provide a list of the available Medicare-certified hospice and SNFs that serve the geographic area requested by the patient. In addition, the discharge plan shall not specify or limit qualified hospice or SNFs and must identify those entities to whom the patient is referred in which the hospital has a disclosable financial interest or in which the HHA has an interest in the hospital.

Therefore, we expect hospitals to provide a list of hospice, HHAs, or SNFs that are available to the patient, that participate in the Medicare program, and that serve the geographic area that the patient requests. The list must be presented only to patients for whom posthospital hospice services, HHA services, or SNF extended care services are indicated and appropriate as determined by the discharge planning evaluation. It is not expected that patients without a need for posthospital hospice services, HHA services, or SNF extended care services would receive the list. The hospital must document in the patient's medical record that a list of hospices, HHAs, or SNFs was presented to the patient or individual acting on the patient's behalf. This serves to document that the requirement was met. Finally, the hospital has the flexibility to develop and maintain its own list of hospices or SNFs, or, in the case of SNFs, simply print a list from the Nursing Home Compare site on the CMS website, *http://www.medicare.gov/,* based on the geographic area that the patient requests.

§482.43(b)(6) - The hospital must include the discharge planning evaluation in the patient's medical record for use in establishing an appropriate discharge plan and must discuss the results of the evaluation with the patient or individual acting on the patient's behalf.

Interpretive Guidelines §482.43(b)(6)

The hospital must demonstrate the development of a discharge plan evaluation for patients in need and then must discuss the results of the evaluation with the patient or individual acting on the patient's behalf. Documentation of these activities is expected.

The discharge plan evaluation is generally found in the clinical notes if there is no dedicated form. The hospital will be expected to document its decision about the need for a plan, document the existence of plans when needed, and indicate what steps were taken to initially implement the plans. Evidence of an ongoing evaluation of the discharge planning needs of the patient is the important factor.

Documented evidence of discussion of the discharge planning evaluation with the patient, if possible, and interested persons should exist in the medical record. Although not mandated by this CoP, it is preferable that the hospital staff seek information from the patient and family to make the discharge planning evaluation as realistic and as viable as possible. The Patients' Rights CoP (§482.13) does provide the patient the right to participate in the development of their plan of care. Discharge planning is considered a part of the plan of care.

§482.43(c) Standard: Discharge Plan

Interpretive Guidelines §482.43(c)

The hospital must ensure that the discharge plan requirements are met.

§482.43(c)(1) - A registered nurse, social worker, or other appropriately qualified personnel must develop, or supervise the development of, a discharge plan if the discharge planning evaluation indicates a need for a discharge plan.

Interpretive Guidelines §482.43(c)(1)

It is a function of the hospital's management to ensure proper supervision of its employees. Existing training and licensing requirements of a registered nurse and social worker in discharge planning are sufficient. "Other appropriately qualified personnel" may include an MD/DO. The hospital should determine who has the requisite knowledge and skills to do the job regardless of how these were acquired. However, because posthospital services and, ultimately, the patient's recovery and quality of life can be affected by the discharge plan, the plan should be supervised by qualified personnel to ensure professional accountability.

The hospital CoP at §482.13(b): Patients' Rights states that "The patient has the right to participate in the development and implementation of his or her plan of care." (CMS views discharge planning as part of the patient's plan of care). "The patient or his/her representative (as allowed under State law) has the right to make informed decisions regarding his/her care" and "The patient's rights include. . .being involved in care planning and treatment."

§482.43(c)(2) In the absence of a finding by the hospital that a patient needs a discharge plan, the patient's physician may request a discharge plan. In such a case, the hospital must develop a discharge plan for the patient.

Interpretive Guidelines §482.43(c)(2)

The physician can make the final decision as to whether a discharge plan is necessary. The hospital will develop a plan if a physician requests one even if the interdisciplinary team had determined one to be unnecessary.

§482.43(c)(2) In the absence of a finding by the hospital that a patient needs a discharge plan, the patient's physician may request a discharge plan. In such a case, the hospital must develop a discharge plan for the patient.

Interpretive Guidelines §482.43(c)(2)

The physician can make the final decision as to whether a discharge plan is necessary. The hospital will develop a plan if a physician requests one even if the interdisciplinary team had determined one to be unnecessary.

§482.43(c)(3) - The hospital must arrange for the initial implementation of the patient's discharge plan.

Interpretive Guidelines §482.43(c)(3)

The hospital is required to arrange for the initial implementation of the discharge plan. This includes arranging for necessary posthospital services and care, and educating patient/family/caregivers/community providers about posthospital care plans.

§482.43(c)(4) - The hospital must reassess the patient's discharge plan if there are factors that may affect continuing care needs or the appropriateness of the discharge plan.

Interpretive Guidelines §482.43(c)(4)

The discharge plan should be initiated as soon as possible after admission. As changes in the patient's condition and needs occur, the discharge plan must be reassessed and updated to address those changes.

§482.43(c)(6) - The hospital must include in the discharge plan a list of HHAs or SNFs that are available to the patient, that are participating in the Medicare program, and that serve the geographic area (as defined by the HHA) in which the patient resides, or in the case of SNFs, in the geographic area requested by the patient. HHAs must request to be listed by the hospital as available.

§482.43(c)(i) - This list must only be presented to patients for whom home healthcare or posthospital extended care services are indicated and appropriate as determined by the discharge planning evaluation.

§482.43(c)(7) The hospital, as part of the discharge planning process, must inform the patient or the patient's family of their freedom to choose among participating Medicare providers of posthospital care services. . . [The hospital, as part of the discharge planning process, must inform the patient or the patient's family of their freedom to choose among participating Medicare providers of posthospital care services and] must, when possible, respect patient and family preferences when they are expressed.

§482.43(c)(8) The discharge plan must identify any HHA or SNF to which the patient is referred in which the hospital has a disclosable financial interest, as specified by the Secretary, and any HHA or SNF that has a disclosable financial interest in a hospital under Medicare. Financial interests that are disclosable under Medicare are determined in accordance with the provisions of Part 420, Subpart C, of this chapter.

§482.43(d) Standard: Transfer or Referral

The hospital must transfer or refer patients, along with necessary medical information, to appropriate facilities, agencies, or outpatient services, as needed, for follow-up or ancillary care.

Interpretive Guidelines §482.43(d)

The hospital must ensure that patients receive proper posthospital care within the constraints of a hospital's authority under state law and within the limits of a patient's right to refuse discharge-planning services. If a patient exercises the right to refuse discharge planning or to comply with a discharge plan, documentation of the refusal is recommended.

"Medical information" may be released only to authorized individuals according to provision

§482.24(b)(3). Examples of necessary information include functional capacity of the patient, requirements for health care services procedures, discharge summary, and referral forms.

"Appropriate facilities" refers to facilities that can meet the patient's assessed needs on a postdischarge basis and that comply with Federal and state health and safety standards.

§483.43(e) Standard: Reassessment

The hospital must reassess its discharge planning process on an on-going basis. The reassessment must include a review of discharge plans to ensure that they are responsive to discharge needs.

Interpretive Guidelines §483.43(e)

The hospital's discharge planning process must be integrated into its QAPI program. The hospital must have a mechanism in place for ongoing reassessment of its discharge planning process. Although specific parameters or measures that would be included in a reassessment are not required, the hospital should ensure the following factors in the reassessment process:

- The time effectiveness of the criteria to identify patients needing discharge plans

- The quality and timeliness for discharge planning evaluations and discharge plans

- The hospital discharge personnel maintain complete and accurate information to advise patients and their representatives of appropriate options

- The hospital has a coordinated discharge planning process that integrates discharge planning with other functional departments, including the quality assurance and utilization review activities of the institution and involves various disciplines

Source: *State Operations Manual.* Appendix A - Survey Protocol, Regulations and Interpretive Guidelines for Hospitals. (Rev. 47, 06-05-09). Retrieved on January 1, 2011 from *http://cms.gov/manuals/Downloads/som107ap_a_hospitals.pdf*

Hospitals With the Highest Readmission Rates, 2010

Hospitals with the Highest Readmission Rates		
Hospital and Location	Total Patients	Readmission Rate
Magee General Hospital, Magee, MS	169	32.4%
Our Lady of the Resurrection Medical Center, Chicago, IL	772	32.4%
Bates County Memorial Hospital, Butler, MO	191	32.3%
Georgiana Hospital, Georgiana, AL	130	32.3%
Holzer Medical Center, Gallipolis, OH	595	32.1%
Perry Community Hospital, Linden, TN	172	32.1%
Kings County Hospital Center, New York	192	32.0%
Lincoln Medical and Mental Health Center, New York	267	32.0%
Russell County Medical Center, Lebanon, VA	177	31.9%
East Orange General Hospital, East Orange, N.J.	494	31.6%
Pleasant Valley Hospital, Point Pleasant, W.V.	409	31.6%
Source: Centers for Medicare and Medicaid Services, July 2010		

Hospitals With the Lowest Readmission Rates, 2010

Hospitals with the Lowest Readmission Rates		
Hospital and Location	Total Patients	Readmission Rate
Baylor Heart and Vascular Hospital, Dallas, TX	323	17.3%
Dixie Regional Medical Center, St. George, Utah	388	18%
Providence Hospital, Mobile, AL	582	18.3%
St. Patrick Hospital, Missoula, MT	359	18.7%
Greenville Memorial Hospital, Greenville, S.C.	1027	18.9%
Portneuf Medical Center, Pocatello, ID	245	18.9%
Presbyterian Hospital, Albuquerque, N.M.	482	19.1%
Sarasota Memorial Hospital, FL	1319	19.2%
McKay-Dee Hospital Center, Ogden, Utah	406	19.3%
Parkview Medical Center, Pueblo, CO	303	19.3%
St. Vincent Heart Center of Indiana, Indianapolis, IN	675	19.3%
Tallahassee Memorial Hospital, FL	544	19.3%
Source: Centers for Medicare and Medicaid Services, July 2010		

CHAPTER 2
Appendix

Physician Payment Schedules..173

Physician Payment Schedules

Medicare Payments for Selected Initial/New Patient E&M Services						
Level Initial	Hospital	Typical Physician Time	Initial Nursing Facility	Typical Physician Time	Assisted Living, New Patient	Typical Physician Time
I	$95.26	30	$85.16	25	$54.49	20
II	$129.18	50	$119.44	35	$79.39	30
III	$189.80	70	$152.64	45	$133.15	45
IV	N/A	N/A	N/A	N/A	$173.57	60
V	N/A	N/A	N/A	N/A	$203.52	75

This table compares the April 1, 2010 average Medicare payments for different levels of initial hospital and initial NF care and for services provided to new patients. It also lists the typical time (in minutes) that a physician would be expected to spend in providing the different types and levels of service.

Medicare Payments for Selected Subsequent/Established Patient E&M Services						
Level Initial	Hospital	Typical Physician Time	Initial Nursing Facility	Typical Physician Time	Assisted Living, New Patient	Typical Physician Time
I	$35.25	15	$40.78	10	$57.01	15
II	$68.92	25	$62.79	15	$88.77	25
III	$98.87	35	$82.99	25	$124.85	40
IV	N/A	N/A	$122.69	35	$179.34	60
V	N/A	N/A	N/A	N/A	N/A	N/A

This table compares average Medicare payment amounts for subsequent hospital and subsequent NF care to established patients.

Ending Hospital Readmissions: A Blueprint for SNFs

CHAPTER 3
Appendix

Reportable Laboratory Values 177

Reportable Laboratory Values

Critical laboratory values are also called "panic," or "alert" values. Most identify conditions needing immediate treatment, and most require immediate correction. Prompt healthcare provider notification is essential. When reporting, it may be helpful to state the lab normal value, followed by the resident's value. Document who was notified, when the notification was made, and any response, such as action, orders, or no orders. Note all verifications of readbacks in your documentation.

The values that follow should be reported to the healthcare provider by phone immediately upon receiving the test results from the lab. You may follow up with a fax copy of the lab report, but since these values suggest potentially acute problems, phone contact must be the primary notification. Most other lab values may be reported on the next business day, but use good judgment and follow physician orders and facility policies. Before contacting the physician for an abnormal lab value, familiarize yourself with the resident's current condition. Have the chart available for comparison with previous values, allergies, and current medications. Primary notification for lab values not listed here can usually be made by fax. Use this listing as a guideline only. Your facility or physicians may use different criteria because of variations in values from one lab to another. If your facility policies vary from the guidelines listed here, facility policies should prevail.

Complete blood count

- WBC > 11,000

- Hemoglobin (Hb) < 10

- Hematocrit < 24

- Platelets < 70,000

Chemistry

- Blood/urea/nitrogen (BUN) > 60 mg/dL

- Calcium (Ca) < 7, > 11 mg/dL

- Chloride < 80, > 120 mmol/L

- Potassium (K) < 3.3, > 5.6 mg/dL

- Sodium (Na) < 125, > 150 mg/dL

- Creatinine > 4

- Bilirubin < 2, > 18mg/dL

- Blood glucose (either by fingerstick in facility or lab draw as part of chemistry)
  > 300 mg/dL in diabetic resident not using sliding-scale insulin
  > 430 mg/dL (or machine registers high) in diabetic resident using sliding-scale insulin
  < 70 mg/dL in diabetic resident
  < 50 mg/dL in nondiabetic resident

Urinalysis

- Abnormal result in resident with signs and symptoms possibly related to urinary tract infection or urosepsis (e.g., fever or hypothermia, burning sensation, pain, altered mental status)

Bacteriology

- Urine culture > 100,000 colony count with symptoms

- All positive cultures > 100,000 colonies (sputum, blood, or skin) if the resident is not already on appropriate antibiotics per sensitivity report

- All positive stools for *Clostridium difficile*

X-ray

- Any new or unsuspected finding (e.g., fracture, pneumonia, CHF)

Drug levels

Drug levels evaluate the therapeutic effectiveness or potential toxicity of a medication. Levels are commonly drawn for drugs such as antibiotics, phenytoin, lithium, warfarin, and digitalis. Definitions that are used for drawing and reporting some tests are:

- Peak - Highest therapeutic concentration

- Trough - Lowest drug concentration

Peak testing is usually drawn:

- 1–2 hours after oral drug administration

- 30–60 minutes after IV drug administration

Trough testing is usually drawn:

- Immediately before drug administration

Reporting Critical Values of Drug Testing

You should report:

- Levels above therapeutic range of any drug

  - Hold next dose

- Use nursing judgment for values below therapeutic range; drugs with potential
  for serious adverse consequences, such as phenytoin or warfarin should be called

- INR > 3

  - Hold warfarin

- PT (in seconds) 3x control value

  - Hold warfarin

- Occasionally, the HCP will order a drug level for potential over-ingestion of a
  drug or to determine whether the resident is experiencing drug toxicity. If so,
  transfer to the acute care hospital is indicated. All of the values listed here
  should be reported promptly. Panic values for selected, common drugs are:

Drug	Critical Value
Acetaminophen	> 150 ug/mL
Amikacin	> 40 ug/mL
Carbamazepine	> 15 ug/mL
Free phenytoin	> 2.0 ug/mL
Gentamicin	> 12 ug/mL
Lidocaine	> 6.0 ug/mL
Lithium	> 2 mmol/L
NAPA	> 30 mg/L
Pentobarbital	> 45 ug/mL

Phenobarbital	> 45 ug/mL
Phenytoin	> 22 ug/mL
Procainamide	> 12 mg/L
Salicylate	> 30.0 mg/dL
Theophylline	> 22 ug/mL
Tobramycin	> 12 ug/mL
Valproic acid	> 150 ug/mL
Vancomycin	> 40 ug/mL

Warfarin Tests

The prothrombin time (protime, PT) test is performed on blood plasma to determine the activity of prothrombin, or clotting factor II, which is part of the coagulation factor assay. Prothrombin time is most commonly used to monitor oral anticoagulant therapy. The normal control value is 11–15 seconds. For good control, the resident's protime is normally maintained between one and a half and two times the normal control.

Excellent guidelines for reporting laboratory values may be downloaded at
http://tinyurl.com/23ejy53

Figure Appendix 3.1	**Recommended Therapeutic Range for Anticoagulation With Coumadin (Warfarin Sodium)**

Prevention and Treatment of Thromboembolism Associated With:	
INR 2.0-3.0	atrial fibrillation
	bioprosthetic heart valves
	pulmonary embolism
	venous thrombosis
INR 2.5-3.5	mechanical heart valves
	postmyocardial infarction

Ending Hospital Readmissions: A Blueprint for SNFs

CHAPTER 4
Appendix

Medication Reconciliation Policy and Procedure............................185

Medication Discrepancy Tool 188

Medication Reconciliation Policy and Procedure

Definition

Medication reconciliation is the process of verifying, clarifying, and reconciling the resident's most current list of medications against the orders from other settings and the current physician orders within 24 hours of admission. Medication reconciliation is done at each admission, transfer, and discharge.

Policy

All residents will have all medications reconciled within 24 hours of admission and transfer. All resident medications should be reconciled within 24 hours of the time of anticipated discharge. The goal of this process is to generate an accurate medication list.

Purpose

Medication reconciliation is an interdisciplinary process between nursing, the healthcare provider, and the pharmacist that compares the resident's most current list of home medications against the hospital orders (if any) and LTCF physician's orders upon admission, transfer, and discharge. If the resident is transferring from one unit to another, the process compares the medications from the source unit with the orders from the receiving unit. Staff must address discrepancies to ensure the medication list is accurate and to decrease the potential for adverse drug events (ADEs) and omissions.

Admission Procedure

1. The nursing staff on the admitting unit will request the prescription bottles from all pharmaceuticals, over-the-counter medications, and nutraceuticals that the resident is taking at home. If obtaining the bottles is not possible, request the most current list of medications the resident has been taking at home, including dosage, frequencies, routes, and data source. Review documentation from the hospital or other facility if the resident was in another care setting. Make a list of all previous medications.

    -   The discontinued medication list must be available in the medical record, but only current medications will be listed on the medication administration record (MAR). If resident is not a reliable source of information, clarify the information with a family caregiver or seek additional data, such as from the community pharmacy or physician caring for the person in the community.

2. After home medications have been listed, give them to a family member to return home. Instruct the resident and family that these medications may not be reordered at the time of discharge. The resident should not take them again unless specifically instructed to do so.

3. Reconcile the medication list to the physician's admission orders and orders from other facilities, as appropriate.

    -   Make a check (✓) on the list next to medications that have been ordered for current use.

    -   Address medications that have not been reordered with the physician or healthcare provider.

4. List all current medications on the MAR. Compare them with the previous lists. Check the dosage and frequency and clarify discrepancies.

Transfer Procedure

1. Upon transfer out of the unit or facility, provide the next service provider with a summary of the resident's current medications.

2. If the resident transfers from one unit to another within the facility, the receiving unit should compare the orders listed on the MAR with the current physician orders. Check for accuracy and clarify discrepancies.

Nonemergency Discharge Procedure

Discharge medication reconciliation involves reviewing the active routine medications at time of discharge compared with the discharge orders, including prescriptions.

1. Ask the physician to write the discharge prescriptions or orders for another care setting.

2. Prepare a list of medications that the resident should take at home.

3. Compare the ordered discharge medications and scripts to the orders to ensure that resident is receiving what is intended at time of discharge.

    *   Use this list for resident and family teaching.

    *   Document medication teaching.

    *   Give the list to the resident at the time of discharge.

4. Document and communicate discharge medication orders to the next service provider when the resident is discharged.

    *   Make a notation on the chart describing transfer of orders.

Medication Discrepancy Tool

Medication Discrepancy Event Description: Complete one form for each discrepancy.

Causes and Contributing Factors: Check all that apply.

Italicized text suggests client's perspective and/or intended meaning

Client Level Discrepancies

❏ Adverse drug reaction or side effects

❏ Intolerance

❏ Did not fill prescription

❏ Did not need prescription

❏ Money/financial barriers

❏ Intentional nonadherence

   ("I was told to take this but I choose not to.")

❏ Unintentional nonadherence (i.e., knowledge deficit)

   ("I don't understand how to take this medication.")

❏ Performance deficit

   ("Maybe someone showed me, but I can't demonstrate to you that I can.")

Systemic Discrepancies

❏ Prescribed with known allergies/intolerances

❏ Conflicting information from different informational sources

   (e.g., *Discharge instructions state one thing and pill bottle says another.*)

❏ Confusion between brand and generic names

❏ Discharge instructions incomplete/inaccurate/illegible

The client cannot read the handwriting or the information is not written in lay terms.

❏ Duplication

(e.g., *Taking multiple drugs with the same action without any rationale.*)

❏ Incorrect dosage

❏ Incorrect quantity

❏ Incorrect label

❏ Cognitive impairment not recognized

❏ No caregiver/need for assistance not recognized

❏ Sight/dexterity limitations not recognized

Resolution

❏ Advised to stop taking/start taking/change administration of medications

❏ Discussed potential benefits and harm that may result from nonadherence

❏ Encouraged client to call PCP/specialist about problem

❏ Encouraged client to schedule an appointment with healthcare provider to discuss problem at next visit

❏ Encouraged client to talk to pharmacist about problem

❏ Addressed performance/knowledge deficit

❏ Provided resource information to facilitate adherence

❏ Other

Ending Hospital Readmissions: A Blueprint for SNFs

CHAPTER 5
Appendix

Quality Improvement Organizations 193

Medicare Part A - MDS Assessment Dates...................................195

Medicare Payment Examples 196

Quality Improvement Organizations

The Centers for Medicare & Medicaid Services (CMS) provide funding for a national network of Quality Improvement Organizations (QIOs). Each state, territory, and the District of Columbia are assigned to a QIO. QIOs are nonregulatory quality improvement partners. Their materials are free and they are not part of the enforcement process. Use them to help you integrate best practices and improve your outcomes!

Although you have a designated QIO for your state, feel free to check others. The QIOs act as a clearinghouse of resource materials developed and collected both nationally and statewide. They provide online resources for quality improvement interventions, including tools, toolkits, presentations, and links to other resources. The QIO community shares resources with each other and with the healthcare providers they serve. Although most QIOs post the same materials, some are unique to the individual area, and the only way to find them is to check the websites. For example, the Kansas QIO has a number of excellent forms, policies, and procedures that were submitted by their facilities and are not available on other QIO websites. The QIO files posted for downloading are in the public domain and are provided for use free of charge. Links to tools outside of QIO website are subject to the host site's copyright policies. QIO phone numbers are listed at *http://tinyurl.com/4ug3cbs*

State Medicare QIOs

Alabama	Alabama Quality Assurance Foundation	*www.aqaf.com*
Alaska	Qualis Health	*www.qualishealth.org*
Arizona	Health Services Advisory Group	*www.hsag.com*
Arkansas	Arkansas Foundation for Medical Care	*www.afmc.org*
California	Health Services Advisory Group	*www.hsag.com*
Colorado	Colorado Foundation for Medical Care	*www.cfmc.org*
Connecticut	Qualidigm	*www.qualidigm.org*
Delaware	Quality Insights of Delaware	*www.qide.org*
District of Columbia	Delmarva Foundation for Medical Care	*www.delmarvafoundation.org*
Florida	Florida Medical Quality Assurance	*www.fmqai.com*
Georgia	Georgia Medical Care Foundation	*www.gmcf.org*

Ending Hospital Readmissions: A Blueprint for SNFs

State Medicare QIOs *(cont.)*

Hawaii	Mountain-Pacific Quality Health Foundation	www.mpqhf.org
Idaho	Qualis Health	www.qualishealth.org
Illinois	Illinois Foundation for Quality Health Care	www.ifqhc.org
Indiana	Health Care Excel	www.hce.org
Iowa	Iowa Foundation for Medical Care	www.internetifmc.com
Kansas	Kansas Foundation for Medical Care	www.kfmc.org
Kansas	Kansas Health Policy Authority	www.khpa.ks.gov
Kentucky	Health Care Excel	www.hce.org
Louisiana	Louisiana Health Care Review	www.lhcr.org
Maine	Northeast Health Care Quality Foundation	www.nhcqf.org
Maryland	Delmarva Foundation for Medical Care	www.delmarva foundation.org
Massachusetts	MassPRO	www.masspro.org
Michigan	Michigan Peer Review Organization	www.mpro.org
Minnesota	Stratis Health	www.stratishealth.org
Mississippi	Mississippi Information and Quality Healthcare	www.iqh.org
Missouri	Primaris	www.primaris.org
Montana	Mountain-Pacific Quality Health Foundation	www.mpqhf.org
Nebraska	CIMRO of Nebraska	www.cimronebraska.org
Nevada	HealthInsight	www.healthinsight.org
New Hampshire	Northeast Health Care Quality Foundation	www.nhcqf.org
New Jersey	Peer Review Organization of New Jersey	www.pronj.org
New Mexico	New Mexico Medical Review Association	www.nmmra.org
New York	IPRO	www.ipro.org
North Carolina	Medical Review of North Carolina	www.mrnc.org
North Dakota	North Dakota Health Care Review	www.ndhcri.org
Ohio	Ohio KePRO	www.ohiokepro.com
Oklahoma	Oklahoma Foundation for Medical Quality	www.ofmq.com
Oregon	Oregon Medical Professional Review Organization (OMPRO)	www.ompro.org
Pennsylvania	Quality Insights of Pennsylvania	www.qipa.org
Puerto Rico	Quality Improvement Professional Research Organization (QIPRO)	www.qipro.org
Rhode Island	Quality Partners of Rhode Island	www.qualitypartnersri.org
South Carolina	Carolina Medical Review	www.mrnc.org
South Dakota	South Dakota Foundation for Medical Care	www.sdfmc.org
Tennessee	Center for Healthcare Quality	www.qsource.org
Texas	Texas Medical Foundation	www.tmf.org
Utah	HealthInsight	www.healthinsight.org
Vermont	Northeast Health Care Quality Foundation	www.nhcqf.org
Virgin Islands	Virgin Islands Medical Institute	www.vimipro.org
Virginia	Virginia Health Quality Center	www.vhqc.org
Washington	Qualis Health	www.qualishealth.org
West Virginia	West Virginia Medical Institute	www.wvmi.org
Wisconsin	MetaStar	www.metastar.com
Wyoming	Mountain-Pacific Quality Health Foundation	www.mpqhf.org
Links to Additional Web Resources: *www.ehdp.com/links/index.htm*		

Medicare Part A – MDS Assessment Dates

MDS	Covered Stay Days (MDS sets payment for these days)	Assessment Reference Date (ARD)*	Grace Days Available
5 day	Days 1–14	1–5	3
14 day	Days 15–30	11–14	5 **
30 day	Days 31–60	21–29	5
60 day	Days 61–90	50–59	5
90 day	Days 91–100	80–89	5

*For Medicare Part A purposes, the assessment reference date (ARD) is used to identify assessments. This is the date listed at A2300 on the MDS. The ARD is the last day staff can collect information for the listed assessment. Changes that are identified after this date cannot be included. In other words, the ARD assessment accurately reflects the resident's condition. The ARD determines the coverage period of each assessment.

**If the 5-day assessment includes the CAAs and care plan, *and* is intended for use as the comprehensive assessment, the facility may use five grace days in which to complete the 14-day assessment. This does not apply if the comprehensive assessment (with CAAs and care plan) is not completed until day 14.

Ending Hospital Readmissions: A Blueprint for SNFs

Medicare Payment Examples

Example Situation	Inpatient or Outpatient	Part A Payment	Part B Payment
You go to the emergency room for treatment and are subsequently admitted with a physician's order.	Inpatient	Emergency department treatment and hospital services	Physician services
You fall and break an arm. You are treated in the emergency room and a cast is applied before you are discharged home.	Outpatient	Nothing	Physician, hospital services (ER time, treatment, x-rays, cast application)
You visit the emergency room with a complaint of chest pain. You are admitted to the hospital for two days for observation.	Outpatient	Nothing	Physician, hospital outpatient services (ER, diagnostics, lab, EKG, observational care)
You are admitted to the hospital for outpatient surgery. Your blood pressure spikes and the physician admits you overnight for blood pressure monitoring. You are discharged the next day.	Outpatient	Nothing	Physician, surgeon, surgical services, diagnostics, observational care

How Hospital Services Affect SNF Coverage	
Example Service	**How SNF is Affected**
You are seen in the emergency room and admitted to the hospital for three days. You are discharged on the fourth day.	Covered on admission to the SNF because the three-day (three midnights) qualifying hospital stay is met
You are seen in the emergency room. You remain there for 24 hours and are subsequently admitted to the hospital for 48 hours before being discharged. You have spent 72 hours at the hospital, including three midnights.	SNF admission is not covered. The 24 hours spent in the emergency room is observational care. This time does not count towards meeting the qualifying stay requirement.

CHAPTER 6

Appendix

Guidelines for Healthcare Provider Notification for
Change of Condition..199

Guidelines for Healthcare Provider Notification
for Change of Condition

General change in status

❑ Change in cognitive/social/functional (ADL) status/change in appetite or any medical condition listed below

Change in vital signs

❑ Temperature > 101°F oral or tympanic, > 102°F rectal

❑ Hypothermia < 95°F oral or tympanic < 96°F rectal or does not register on thermometer

❑ Increase in respiratory rate; respirations ≥ 24/minute

❑ Decrease in pulse rate; pulse > 100/minute or < 60/minute

Emergency healthcare provider notification

❑ Worsening or unstable vital signs accompanied by hypotension, hypertension, lethargy, decreased oral intake, chills

Routine healthcare provider notification

❑ Symptoms not responding to nursing measures, present for at least 12 hours

❑ Abnormal urinalysis values (fax first; follow up by phone within two hours)

Fever

Emergency healthcare provider notification

❏ New onset fever of > 100°F accompanied by hypotension, hypertension

_____ Temperature > 101°F oral or tympanic, > 102°F rectal

_____ Hypothermia < 95°F oral or tympanic, < 96°F rectal or does not register on thermometer

_____ Increase in respiratory rate; respirations ≥ 24/minute

_____ Increase in pulse rate; pulse > 100/minute

AND/OR
One or more of the following:

❏ Profound lethargy

❏ Decreased oral intake

❏ Chills

❏ Glucose > 300

Routine healthcare provider notification

❏ Fever, not responding to nursing measures, present for at least 12 hours

Change in cognitive or functional status

❏ New onset lethargy

❏ New onset change in mental status

Urinary tract signs and symptoms:

_____ Change in urine

❑ Frequency

❑ Urgency

❑ Color

❑ Clarity

❑ Odor

Emergency healthcare provider notification

❑ Worsening symptoms accompanied by hypotension, hypertension, lethargy, decreased oral intake, chills

Routine healthcare provider notification

❑ Symptoms not responding to nursing measures, present for at least 12 hours

❑ Abnormal urinalysis values (fax first; follow up by phone within two hours)

Respiratory signs and symptoms:

_____ New or swollen/tender glands in the neck

_____ Onset of upper respiratory symptoms

❑ Nasal congestion and/or drainage appearance _____

❑ Runny nose

❑ Sneezing

❑ Sore throat

Ending Hospital Readmissions: A Blueprint for SNFs

❏ Cough ___ productive ___ nonproductive

❏ Rhonchi

❏ Crackles (rales, crepitations)

❏ Wheezes

❏ Bronchial breathing

❏ Pleuritic chest pain

or

_____ Onset of flu-like illness symptoms

❏ Chills

❏ Headache

❏ Eye pain

❏ Malaise

❏ Muscle aches

or

_____ Onset of other lower respiratory symptoms

❏ New/increase cough or sputum

❏ New shortness of breath (SOB)

❏ Inceased respiratory rate

Emergency healthcare provider notification

❑ Dyspnea or SOB not promptly relieved by nursing measures and/or PRN medication.

❑ Sudden drop in pulse oximeter. ≤ 90% suggests an impending crisis; < 85% indicates hypoxemia; < 70% indicates a life threatening condition.

Routine healthcare provider notification

❑ Worsening condition

❑ No improvement within 72 hours of a change in physician orders for this condition

❑ Need for initial PRN orders

Gastrointestinal (GI) signs and symptoms:

_____ Onset of two or more episodes of watery stools within a 24-hour period

_____ Onset of two or more episodes of vomiting within a 24-hour period

_____ Flank or suprapubic pain or tenderness

_____ Abdominal pain/tenderness

Emergency healthcare provider notification

❑ New, acute gastrointestinal symptom accompanied by hypotension, hypertension, profound lethargy, decreased oral intake, and/or chills

Routine healthcare provider notification

❑ GI symptoms not responding to nursing measures; present and/or worsening over several hours

Skin/soft tissue signs and symptoms:

_____ New purulent drainage

_____ Redness

_____ Pain/tenderness

_____ Heat/warmth is present at a wound, skin, or soft tissue site

Emergency healthcare provider notification

❏ Sudden onset of significant facial and/or neck edema

Routine healthcare provider notification

❏ Worsening condition or no improvement within 48-hour period of order change

❏ Need to obtain initial and/or PRN orders

Lower Respiratory Bacterial Infection

Three or more of the following:

❏ New/increased cough

❏ New/increased sputum

❏ Fever

❏ Change in cognitive/functional status

❏ New crackles (rales), rhonchi, wheezes

❏ Bronchial breathing, OR

One or more of:

❏ New SOB

❏ Increased respiratory rate > 24/min

❏ Change in cognitive/functional status (see values above)

Emergency healthcare provider notification

❏ Dyspnea or SOB not promptly relieved by nursing measures and/or PRN medication

❏ Sudden drop in pulse oximeter (see values on previous page)

Routine healthcare provider notification

❏ worsening condition

❏ no improvement within 72 hours of a change in physician orders for this condition

❏ need for initial PRN orders

Upper Respiratory Bacterial Infection

Two or more of:

❏ Runny nose or sneezing

❏ Stuffy nose (nasal congestion)

❏ Sore throat/hoarseness/difficulty swallowing

❏ Dry cough

❏ New swollen or tender glands in the neck (cervical lymphadenopathy)

Emergency healthcare provider notification

❏ Dyspnea or SOB not promptly relieved by nursing measures and/or PRN medication

❏ Sudden drop in pulse oximeter

Routine healthcare provider notification

❏ Worsening condition

❏ No improvement within 72 hours of a change in physician orders for this condition

❏ Need for initial PRN orders

Symptomatic Urinary Tract Infection: Resident Without Indwelling Catheter

Three or more of the following:

❏ Fever or chills

❏ New burning pain or frequency or urgency on urination

❏ Flank or suprapubic pain or tenderness

❏ Change in character of urine

❏ Change in cognitive status

❏ Change in functional status

❏ New or worsening incontinence

❏ Lethargy

Symptomatic Urinary Tract Infection: Resident With Indwelling Catheter

Two or more of the following:

❑ Fever or chills

❑ Flank or suprapubic pain or tenderness

❑ Change in character of urine

❑ Change in cognitive status

❑ Change in functional status

❑ Lethargy

Emergency healthcare provider notification

❑ Worsening symptoms accompanied by hypotension, hypertension, lethargy, decreased oral intake, chills

Routine healthcare provider notification

❑ Symptoms not responding to nursing measures; present for at least 12 hours

❑ Abnormal urinalysis values (fax first; follow up by phone within two hours)

Skin/Soft Tissue Infection

One or more of the following:

❑ Pus (purulent drainage) present at a wound, skin, or soft tissue site

❑ Positive culture and sensitivity

Emergency healthcare provider notification

❑ Sudden onset of significant facial and/or neck edema.

Routine healthcare provider notification

❑ Worsening condition or no improvement within 48-hour period of order change

❑ Need to obtain initial and/or PRN orders

Four or more of the following:

❑ Fever

❑ Worsening cognitive/functional status

And/or, at the site of infection, new or increased:

❑ Heat

❑ Redness

❑ Swelling

❑ Tenderness

❑ Serous drainage

Emergency healthcare provider notification

❑ Sudden onset of significant facial and/or neck edema

Routine healthcare provider notification

❑ Worsening condition or no improvement within 48-hour period of order change

❑ Need to obtain initial and/or PRN orders

Suspected Infection: Site Unknown

Documentation in the medical record:

❏ Fever (as previously defined) on two or more occasions at least 12 hours apart in any three day period

and

❏ Absence of any of the criteria in the previously listed sites

Chest Pain

Emergency healthcare provider notification

❏ Chest pain, unrelieved by nitroglycerine x 3 (NTG x 3), should be reported as an emergency

❏ New onset or recurrence of chest pain not relieved by NTG x 3

❏ Significant change in vital signs

❏ Fingerstick blood sugar > 300

Routine healthcare provider notification

❏ Chest pain, relieved by NTG, and

❏ Status and/or vital signs have not returned to baseline

❏ Increased use of PRN NTG in short interval

Follow-up/Ongoing Notifications for Chest Pain

Emergency healthcare provider notification

❑ Dyspnea or SOB not promptly relieved by nursing measures and/or PRN medication

❑ Sudden drop in pulse oximeter (see previously listed values)

Routine healthcare provider notification

❑ Worsening condition

❑ No improvement within 72 hours of a change in physician orders for this condition

❑ Need for initial PRN orders

Falls and Fractures or Injuries

Emergency healthcare provider notification

For lacerations or wounds with the following:

❑ Deep, long, or irregular shaped lacerations

❑ Bleeding profusely, which cannot be stopped with ice and pressure

❑ Facial wounds ≥ 1cm

❑ Foreign body present in wound

❑ Apparent fracture with angulation of extremity or obvious compound fracture

❑ Sudden loss of color, warmth, or feeling in hand or foot of injured extremity

❑ Loss of consciousness > 3 minutes

❑ Extreme blood pressure change lasting > 30 minutes

Routine healthcare provider notification

❑ Incident without change in vital signs but with pain or dysfunction lasting ≥
1 hour

Healthcare Provider Notification for Any Change in Condition

Emergency healthcare provider notification

❑ Sudden onset of significant status change especially with neurological changes

❑ Any significant change in mental status

❑ Any significant change in vital signs

❑ New onset lethargy

❑ New onset hypotension

❑ New onset hypertension

❑ New onset fever ≥ 101°F oral or tympanic or ≥ 102°F rectal

Routine healthcare provider notification

❑ Worsening condition or no improvement within 48-hour period of change
in orders

❑ Need to obtain initial and/or PRN orders

Use good nursing judgment in calling the healthcare provider. Review the resident's chart over the past few days so you have an idea of the resident's condition and status.

Ending Hospital Readmissions: A Blueprint for SNFs

Complete a focused assessment of the resident's condition before placing the call. If a problem does not fit into any of the previous categories and you feel it warrants healthcare provider notification and/or orders, place the call and report the resident's signs and symptoms as well as the results of your focused nursing assessment. The documentation guidelines in *Clinical Documentation: An Essential Guide for Long Term Care* Nurses will be useful to you in determining what to assess. This book is available at *www.hcmarketplace.com/prod 4923.html*

Be prepared to inform the healthcare provider with every phone call if the resident is:

- Diabetic

- On dialysis

- On warfarin or other anticoagulants

If the resident has any of these conditions, have the chart available and be prepared to report recent laboratory reports; medication to treat the condition, the dosage, and frequency; and recent fingerstick blood sugars if the resident is a diabetic.

Nursing Action After Healthcare Provider Notification

❑ Licensed nurse reviews and implements new orders from healthcare provider

❑ Orders medication from pharmacy

❑ Orders lab

❑ Updates plan of care

❑ Notifies responsible party

❏ Flags record for follow-up assessment and charting every shift

    – Document your assessment of the condition for which antibiotics are being given. Lack of side effects to antibiotics is secondary.

❏ Flags record for vital signs every shift (every four hours if abnormal)

Examples of Change in Condition Reporting to an Healthcare Provider

The conditions listed here are examples only. Use good nursing judgment and the results of your complete assessment when making the determination about whether to call the healthcare provider immediately or the next business day. Document all attempts, notifications, readbacks, orders, and responses from the healthcare provider and interested family members who were also notified. If the resident's condition worsens after notifying the healthcare provider, call again. If the primary healthcare provider is not available, notify the healthcare provider on call. If this person is not available, contact the facility medical director, or follow facility policies for making notifications. Residents with the following conditions must be monitored (including vital signs and focused system assessments) by nursing personnel every shift until the condition has been eliminated or stabilized for at least 24 hours. When these conditions are identified, use resident PRN orders, facility standing orders or protocols, and nursing measures to treat them.

Also see Vital Signs Suggesting an Acute Change in Condition. Additional information is available at:

- *http://tinyurl.com/62juyr3*

- *http://tinyurl.com/66pgeun*

- *http://tinyurl.com/69n9ala*

Figure Appendix 6.1

Condition, Nursing Diagnosis	Immediate Reporting	Report Next Office Day
Anxiety	Acute confusion, new onset change in mental status, crying, situation intolerable for resident	Anxious, restless, intermittent crying
Bleeding	Resident is on warfarin or another anticoagulant. Uncontrolled, heavy, or recurrent, need for sutures, nosebleeds, gross blood in emesis, urine, stools, vaginal drainage, etc.	Controlled bleeding, small amount of bleeding, no recurrence, managed and contained with nursing measures
Breathing pattern, ineffective	Sudden onset, change in vital signs, accompanied by chest pain, cyanosis or color change, breathing labored	May be recurrent but resident is not in acute distress and obtains at least partial relief from PRN orders and nursing measures, no change in vital signs, color adequate
Chest pain	New onset, recurrent pain not relieved by NTG x 3 doses in 20 minutes. Chest pain accompanied by SOB, change in vitals, diaphoresis, emesis	History of chest pain that responds to nursing measures, including NTG PRN, if ordered
Combative behavior	Resident on new medication, sudden onset change in mental status, behavior does not respond to nursing care, is a danger to self or others	Mild or recurrent combativeness
Confusion, acute	Sudden onset	Gradual, progressive onset
Constipation	Rigid or distended abdomen, pain, no bowel sounds, no treatment ordered and resident in distress	Not responding to PRN regimen and nursing measures, resident has had two or more episodes in past 30 days
Coping, ineffective	Expresses suicidal intent; resident has the abilty and/or means to carry out threat, need for prompt mental health interventions	Responding to suicide precautions initiated by facility, chronic depression or sadness, no specific suicide plan
Diarrhea (three loose stools in 24 hours or use facility definition)	Acute onset, accompanied by severe abdominal pain, vomiting, or other symptoms, change in vital signs, change in mental status	Recurrent or persistent loose stools, stable vital signs

Ending Hospital Readmissions: A Blueprint for SNFs

(cont.)

Condition, Nursing Diagnosis	Immediate Reporting	Report Next Office Day
Emesis, vomiting	Frank blood or coffee grounds, change in vital signs, persistent vomiting, not responding to nursing measures	Single emesis managed by nursing measures, stable vital signs
Enteral feeding tube	Tube is plugged, removed, etc. and cannot be reinserted ; potential aspiration or signs/symptoms of peritonitis	Signs of feeding intolerance, vomiting, leakage at insertion site, tube has been removed and nurse can replace using a PRN order
Eye pain or discomfort	Change in vision, complains of seeing halos, sudden onset severe/ unremitting eye pain	Minor itching or discomfort that responds at least partially to PRN orders, nursing measures, and comfort measures such as warm or cool compresses
Fall(s)	Need for sutures, head injury, obvious deformity, inability to use injured extremity, abnormal neuro checks, uncontrolled bleeding	No injury or minor injury that responds to nursing measures and PRN orders
Family request, resident request	Insistent, demanding that physician be contacted	Family has observed a minor or persistent problem and wants physician informed
Fluid volume, deficient fluid volume, risk for deficient	Fluid intake 50% of usual in past 24 hours, vomiting, or diarrhea, change in mental status, abnormal vital signs, abnormal labs	Not responding to nursing interventions, vital signs and mental status within normal limits for resident
Fluid volume, excess edema	Acute onset, edema in one leg, tenderness, redness, shortness of breath, unable to palpate pulse in extremity, change in vital signs	Recurrent edema, or increased size of existing edema, gradual weight gain, stable vital signs
Hyperthermia (temperature > 100° F oral or tympanic, > 101°F rectal)	Worsening or unstable vital signs accompanied by hypotension, hypertension, chills, increase in respiratory rate; respirations $\geq$ 24/minute, increase in pulse rate; pulse >100/minute, lethargy, change in mental status, decreased fluid intake, elevated blood glucose	Symptoms not responding to nursing measures, present for at least 12 hours; abnormal urinalysis values (fax first; follow up by phone within two hours)

Ending Hospital Readmissions: A Blueprint for SNFs

(cont.)

Figure Appendix 6.1

Condition, Nursing Diagnosis	Immediate Reporting	Report Next Office Day
Hypothermia (temperature < 95° F oral or tympanic, < 96°F rectal or does not register on thermometer)	Worsening or unstable vital signs accompanied by hypotension, hypertension, lethargy, decreased oral intake, chills, increase in respiratory rate; respirations ≥ 24/minute, increase in pulse rate; pulse > 100/minute, lethargy, change in mental status, decreased fluid intake, chills, elevated blood glucose	Symptoms not responding to nursing measures, present for at least 12 hours; abnormal urinalysis values (fax first; follow up by phone within two hours)
Medication error	Resident is symptomatic, resident needs treatment such as Narcan; error is significant (such as giving insulin to a nondiabetic)	Resident is stable and asymptomatic, insignificant error
Pain, acute	New injury or medical problem, new or sudden onset pain, no PRN order or PRN is ineffective, resident rates pain as ≥ 4 on a 10 point scale, abnormal vital signs	Pain partially relieved by an existing PRN order and is tolerable to resident
Pulse, change in pulse rate (pulse > 100/minute or < 60/minute)	Worsening or unstable vital signs accompanied by hypotension, hypertension, lethargy, decreased oral intake, chills	Symptoms not responding to nursing measures, present for at least 12 hours; abnormal urinalysis values (fax first; follow up by phone within two hours)
Rash	Probable allergic reaction, hives, swelling in face and neck, resident taking new medication, uncontrolled pruritus, signs of respiratory distress, hypotension	Minor rash, controlled by nursing measures and PRN orders, localized or recurrent rash tolerable to resident
Respirations, increase in respiratory rate (respirations ≥ 24/minute)	Worsening or unstable vital signs accompanied by hypotension, hypertension, lethargy, decreased oral intake, chills	Symptoms not responding to nursing measures, present for at least 12 hours; abnormal urinalysis values (fax first; follow up by phone within two hours)

Figure Appendix 6.1 **(cont.)**

Condition, Nursing Diagnosis	Immediate Reporting	Report Next Office Day
Seizure(s)	New onset, recurrent or continuous seizures, status epilepticus, seizure does not stop after several minutes, abnormal vital signs, unable to administer PRN for seizure activity, responsiveness does not return following seizure	Known history of seizures, limited seizure that does not recur, resident on antiseizure medication
Self-care deficit	Abnormal vital signs or neurological deficit, acute confusion/change in mental status	Progressive deterioration in self-care ability, gradually increasing confusion
Skin integrity, impaired	Laceration or injury needing sutures, Stage II, III, IV pressure ulcer with no treatment order	Injury responds to nursing measures and existing orders, new Stage I ulcer, increase in size or other problem with existing ulcers
Suicide, risk for	Expresses suicidal intent; resident has the abilty and/or means to carry out threat, need for prompt mental health interventions	Responding to suicide precautions initiated by facility, chronic depression or sadness, no specific suicide plan
Urinary retention	Resident unable to void, bladder distention, increasing discomfort, elevated temp or hypothermia, change in mental status	No bladder distention, resident feels as if he or she is not emptying completely, has urgency and other signs of UTI, afebrile or low-grade temp
Urinary tract abnormalities (suspected infection) change in urine, (i.e., frequency, urgency, color, clarity, odor)	Worsening symptoms accompanied by hypotension, hypertension, lethargy, decreased oral intake, chills, fever, hypothermia	Symptoms not responding to nursing measures, present for at least 12 hours, abnormal urinalysis values (fax first; follow up by phone within two hours)
Wandering	Resident has eloped or has gotten out of facility despite staff's best efforts to contain him or her	Resident went outside, but was returned promptly by staff without injury

Ending Hospital Readmissions: A Blueprint for SNFs

Pulse Assessment and Documentation

Normal pulse ranges from approximately 60–100 BPM, but this can vary by about 10%. The following clinical presentations may indicate an acute condition change and should be assessed further:

- Sustained change from normal range

- Change in usual pulse rhythm or regularity

- Pulse > 120 BPM or < 50 BPM (use facility criteria; many facilities use > 100 or < 60)

- Pulse > 100 BPM combined with other symptoms (e.g., palpitations, dyspnea, dizziness)

Note whether pulses are:

- Strong

- Weak

- Absent

- Equal (†) Bilaterally

- > on Right

- > on Left

- Pulse Assessment

  - Peripheral: Identify pulse rhythm, volume, and rate

  - Apical: Listen with the diaphragm of stethoscope

- Locate apex of heart, usually at the left fifth intercostal at the midclavicular line

    - Note strength and regularity of rhythm

    - Count rate (count one full minute if the rhythm is irregular)

Pulse Oximetry Values

The pulse oximetry value is considered the fifth vital sign in many facilities. Hemoglobin carries oxygen to nourish the cells. The pulse oximeter measures the level of saturation of the resident's hemoglobin with oxygen. The pulse oximeter measures how full the hemoglobin molecules are with oxygen. The measurement may be done continuously or intermittently. The pulse oximeter often detects critical changes in the resident's oxygen levels before the skin color changes or other signs and symptoms are evident, making it a valuable tool. Using the pulse oximeter will provide information immediately when changes occur. The resident's outcome is usually better when early treatment is provided. Before applying the pulse oximeter, check the resident's oxygen, if used. Make sure the oxygen liter flow is set as ordered by the physician. Document the liter flow. Also note and document the resident's baseline values taken at the time the pulse oximeter is applied:

- Vital signs.

- Initial oxygen saturation reading.

- Note the resident's pulse rate, if the unit provides this reading. Compare with the resident's actual pulse to make sure the unit is picking up each beat.

- Monitor the resident's respirations and general appearance.

- Note the resident's color.

- If abnormal values are noted, document your focused assessment of the resident's condition at the time the abnormal value is noted.

Signs and symptoms of decreased ability to ventilate are:

- Capillary refill > 3 seconds.

- Cyanosis.

- Dyspnea.

- Tachypnea.

- Decreased level of consciousness.

- Increased work of breathing.

- Decreasing ability to protect airway.

- Monitor the resident, not the machine; if the unit shows life-threatening values but the resident is in no distress, reconcile the problem. Document focused assessment and vital signs.

Figure Appendix 6.2

Pulse Oximeter Reading	Interpretation
95%–100%	Normal
Below 90%	Suggests complications, impending hypoxemia
85%	Inadequate oxygen for body function, condition worsening, potential impending crisis
Below 70%	Life-threatening

Vital Signs Suggesting an Acute Change in Condition

Temperature

- A range of 98.2°F (36.8°C) to 99.9°F (37.7°C) oral temperature is considered normal. A resident's normal temperature will vary by up to 0.9°F (0.5°C) daily.

- Try to establish the resident's normal temperature range as soon as possible after admission. This can be readily done if regular admission monitoring includes vital signs. Consider taking vital signs every shift (or more often if abnormal) during this assessment period.

- A sudden or rapid change from normal temperature may suggest an acute change of condition. One temperature reading above 100°F, two readings above 99°F, or an increase of 2°F above the upper end of the resident's normal range may be a positive sign of an acute condition change.

- After an isolated temperature reading that is outside the resident's normal range, repeat temperature readings approximately every four hours for 24 hours and assess for other signs and symptoms to determine whether an acute change of condition exists.

- Hypothermia may also indicate a possible acute change of condition. Subnormal temperatures often indicate acute illness or shock in elderly persons.

- An electric thermometer is the preferred method for taking temperature. Avoid the axillary method unless other methods are contraindicated. If a tympanic thermometer is used, make sure the lens is inserted correctly and is flat against the eardrum.

- Assess the resident for factors that may affect temperature, such as medications.

Pulse

Normal pulse ranges from approximately 60–100 BPM, but this can vary by about 10%. The following clinical presentations may indicate an acute condition change and should be assessed further:

- Sustained change from normal range

- Change in usual pulse rhythm or regularity

- Pulse >120 BPM or < 50 BPM (use facility criteria; many facilities use >100 or < 60)

- Pulse >100 BPM combined with other symptoms (e.g., palpitations, dyspnea, dizziness)

Note and document whether pulses are:

- Strong

- Weak

- Absent

- Equal (†) Bilaterally

- > on Right

- > on Left

- Pulse assessment

  - Peripheral: Identify pulse rhythm, volume, and rate

  - Apical: Listen with the diaphragm of stethoscope

- Locate apex of heart, usually at the left fifth intercostal at the midclavicular line

  – Note strength and regularity of rhythm

  – Count rate (count one full minute if the rhythm is irregular)

Nursing assessment of pulse strength

4 = Bounding

3 = Full, increased

2 = Normal

1 = Diminished, barely palpable

0 = Absent

Grading pulses

0 = Absent pulse

1 + = Pulse is weak and/or thready (commonly due to dehydration, decreased volume, or blood pressure)

2 + = Normal

3 + = Full (commonly caused by fever or exercise)

4 + = Full and bounding (almost always abnormal, suggests excessive circulating volume or hypertension)

Respirations

Observe the resident for the following signs and symptoms:

- Respiratory rates > 28 breaths/min (younger adults: 12–15 breaths/min; elderly: 16–25 breaths/min; with approximate 2:1 inspiration/expiration ratio)

- Marked change from usual respiration pattern or rhythm

- Irregular breathing, long pauses between breaths, audible noises related to breathing

- Struggling to breathe (e.g., gasping for breath, using accessory muscles of the neck)

- Pulse oximetry values, < 90

- Capillary refill, > 3 seconds

Blood pressure

- Try to establish the resident's usual blood pressure (B/P) range as soon as possible after admission. This can be readily done if regular admission monitoring includes vital signs. Consider taking vital signs every shift (or more often if abnormal) during this assessment period. (Normal range is approximately systolic 100–140 mmHg, diastolic 60–90 mmHg. Note: New criteria were released in 2003 that further divide the normal category. For additional information, see *http://www.nhlbi.nih.gov/hbp/*)

- A change in B/P is more often a symptom than a cause of an acute change of condition. Isolated B/P elevations generally are not significant. Sustained elevations in systolic pressure should trigger further assessment. A B/P change alone should not trigger a call to the practitioner without additional signs or symptoms (e.g., sustained elevation, new neurological symptoms). Complete a focused assessment to identify the cause.

- A decrease in systolic B/P > 120 mmHg when moving from a prone to a seated position or from a standing position signals orthostatic hypotension. This condition is a great contributing risk factor for falls and is often overlooked. Consult the healthcare provider, if the condition is identified. Note on care plan and fall risk documentation.

- Any significant decrease in B/P may signal an acute change of condition (e.g., systolic B/P < 100 mmHg if baseline is 110 mmHg, decline in B/P accompanied by other symptoms such as dizziness, decline > 15 mm in systolic B/P, combination of pulse > 100 BPM and/or systolic B/P < 100 mmHg.

- If abnormal values noted, document your focused assessment of the resident's condition at the time the abnormal value is noted.

Signs and symptoms of decreased ability to ventilate are:

- Capillary refill >3 seconds

- Cyanosis

- Dyspnea

- Tachypnea

- Decreased level of consciousness

- Increased work of breathing

- Decreasing ability to protect airway

Monitor the resident, not the machine; if the unit shows life-threatening values but the resident is in no distress, reconcile the problem. Document focused assessment and vital signs.

General guidelines for abnormal vital sign reporting

- If the resident is symptomatic, follow guidelines for immediate reporting. Use good nursing judgment when determining whether to report immediately or wait until next business day.

Ending Hospital Readmissions: A Blueprint for SNFs

- All vital signs in the immediate and next day reporting category must be monitored every four hours or as ordered until they have been stable for 72 hours.

Guidelines for immediate reporting

- Pulse oximeter below 90

- Systolic B/P > 210 mmHg, < 90 mmHg

- Diastolic B/P > 115 mmHg

- Resting pulse > 130 BPM, < 55 BMP, or > 110 BPM and patient has dyspnea or palpitations

- Respirations > 28, s < 10/minute

- Oral (electronic thermometer) temperature > 101°F

- Oral (electronic thermometer) temperature < 96° F

Guidelines for reporting next business day

- Diastolic B/P routinely > 90 mmHg

- Resting pulse > 120 BPM on repeat exam

- Oral (electronic thermometer) temperature > 100°F

- Oral (electronic thermometer) temperature < 97° F

CHAPTER 7

Appendix

Assessment and Documentation Guidelines for
Congestive Heart Failure...229

Assessment and Documentation Guidelines for
Myocardial Infarction...232

Survey Audit Checklist 235

Transition Coordinator Job Description 248

Assessment and Documentation Guidelines for Congestive Heart Failure

Definitions

- **Heart failure:** The inability of the heart to pump blood to the body parts sufficient to meet metabolic demands.

Types

- **Acute heart failure:** Sudden onset of inability of the heart to contract; may cause life-threatening signs and symptoms, including pulmonary edema.

- **Chronic heart failure:** Compromise in the ability of the heart to pump efficiently; often occurs as a result of another chronic disorder. When a resident has chronic heart failure, he or she develops signs and symptoms of both right-sided and left-sided heart failure.

- **Congestive heart failure (CHF):** An accumulation of blood and fluid in tissues and organs from impaired circulation.

Assess and document the following each shift:

- Vital signs

- Capillary refill

- Initiate pulse oximetry

- Check for and consider recent laboratory values, if any

- Evaluate new medications and side effects, if any

- Monitor for signs/symptoms dehydration and inadequate fluid intake (which causes hypovolemia)

  – Consider intake and output (I & O) monitoring

- Note any other changes from resident's usual condition (what he or she is like on a normal day)

- If resident on warfarin, review and report most recent prothrombin (PT) and International Normalized Ratio (INR), coagulation status, signs of internal bleeding

Right-sided heart failure

- Ascites

- Nausea and/or vomiting

- Weight gain (gradual)

- Jugular venous distention

- Weakness

- Edema, fluid retention

- Rings, shoes, clothing seem tight as edema progresses

- Dependent pitting edema in feet and ankles

- Edema may disappear at night but recurs when up

- Dysrhythmias

- Enlarged abdominal organs

Left-sided heart failure

- Unusual fatigue with minimal activity

- Exertional dyspnea

- Hypoxia

- Orthopnea

- Paroxysmal nocturnal dyspnea

- Fatigue

- Cyanosis

- Crackles

- Cough

- Expectorates pink, frothy sputum

- Rapid, irregular pulse

- Elevated blood pressure

- Decreased urine output

- Progressive restlessness and confusion

- Anorexia

- Nausea

- Flatulence

Adapted from: Acello, Barbara. (2007.) *Clinical Documentation: An Essential Guide for Long Term Care Nurse*, HCPro Inc. *www.hcmarketplace.com/prod-4923/Clinical-Documentation.html*

Assessment and Documentation Guidelines
for Myocardial Infarction

Myocardial infarction

- Check for and consider recent laboratory values, if any

- Evaluate new medications and side effects, if any

- Note any other changes from resident's usual condition (what he or she is like on a normal day)

- If resident on warfarin, review and report most recent prothrombin time (PT) and International Normalized Ratio (INR), coagulation status, signs of internal bleeding

Assess and document the following each shift:

- Vital signs

- Capillary refill

- Initiate pulse oximetry

- Sudden onset severe chest pain

- Pain usually substernal; may radiate to shoulder, arm, teeth, jaw, or throat

- Apprehension/anxiety

- Pallor

- Diaphoresis

- Hypotension

- Rapid, weak, and/or irregular pulse

- Feeling faint

- Nausea and/or vomiting

- May have dyspnea, cyanosis, cough

- Fever, abnormal vital signs

Chest pain

Chest pain is a serious medical emergency. When a resident reports chest pain, perform the following:

- Check the vital signs.

- Capillary refill.

- Initiate pulse oximetry.

- Notify the healthcare provider.

- Provide oxygen at 3 liters/minute per cannula. Increase according to degree of resident's distress, cyanosis, etc.

- Complete a quick physical assessment, including heart and lung sounds.

- Check peripheral pulses bilaterally.

- Check blood pressure in both arms.

- Assess for trauma, edema, and bleeding

After your initial interventions, use the PQRST mnemonic to obtain additional information:

P = Provoked or palliative

- What caused or preceded the chest pain? What was the resident doing (activity) when the pain began?

Q = Quality

- Provide a description of the pain (e.g., crushing, stabbing, like an elephant standing on the chest). Use the resident's words in quotes.

R = Region and radiation

- Where did the pain begin? Does it radiate? If so, to where? It may be helpful to instruct the resident to point to a specific spot. Otherwise the resident gesture the entire chest.

S = Severity of pain

- Ask the resident to rate the pain on a scale of 1 to 10, with 1 being the least and 10 being the most painful.

T = Time

- Ask the resident to state what time the pain began and describe the duration.

Adapted from Acello, Barbara. (2007.) *Clinical Documentation: An Essential Guide for Long Term Care Nurses,* HCPro, Inc. *www.hcmarketplace.com/prod-4923/Clinical-Documentation.html*

Ending Hospital Readmissions: A Blueprint for SNFs

Survey Audit Checklist

Stage II—Critical Elements for Rehabilitation and Community Discharge

Facility Name: _____ Facility ID: _____ Date: _____

Surveyor Name: _____

Resident Name: _____ Resident ID: _____

Initial Admission Date: _____ Interviewable: ❑ Yes ❑ No Resident Room: _____

Care Area(s): _____

Use

For a resident:
- ❑ Admitted for rehabilitation, received PT, OT, or ST services but was not discharged back to the community (may have been discharged to another long-term care facility/skilled nursing facility); or
- ❑ Whose most recent MDS (5 and 14 day comparison) assessments indicates the resident received PT or OT but did not improve in transferring ability.

NOTE: Although this review is triggered by lack of improvement in transfer ability, all areas of functional ability should be reviewed, as pertinent to the individual. Use to determine whether the facility provided care to ensure that (a) the resident received necessary rehabilitative services and, (b) based on discharge potential, discharge planning was provided.

Procedure

- ❑ Briefly review the assessment, care plan, and orders to identify facility interventions and to guide observations to be made.
- ❑ Corroborate observations by interview and record review.

Ending Hospital Readmissions: A Blueprint for SNFs

Observations	
❑ Observe whether staff consistently implement the care plan over time and across various shifts. Staff are expected to assess and provide appropriate care from the day of admission. During observations of interventions, note and/or follow up on deviations from the care plan, deviations from current standards of practice, as well as potential negative outcomes. Determine whether: ❑ The resident received encouragement and needed assistance to perform therapy tasks (while in therapy sessions). ❑ Nursing staff provided restorative nursing services to foster improvement in functioning in accordance with the treatment plan such as assisting the resident to walk with a gait belt as planned. assisting the resident to button rather than doing it for them, and assisting the resident to use communication devices. ❑ The resident was provided supportive and assistive devices/equipment as assessed, received encouragement and assistance to use the device(s) on a regular basis, and that devices fit properly. ❑ The resident exhibits signs of pain during treatment sessions, and whether staff intervene or address the pain. ❑ The resident is afforded privacy during treatments that expose the body.	**Notes:**

Resident/Representative Interview	
Interview the resident, family, or responsible party as appropriate to identify: ❑ The resident's/representative's involvement in the development of the care plan, defining the approaches and goals, and whether interventions reflect choice and preferences. ❑ The resident's/representative's awareness of the interventions in use and how to use devices or equipment. ❑ Whether the resident comprehends and applies information and instructions to help improve functioning. ❑ Whether staff allows the resident sufficient time to perform rehabilitative and restorative tasks. ❑ The presence of pain that affects ability to make rehabilitative progress; including location, cause, and how it is managed. ❑ If interventions are refused, whether alternatives were offered. ❑ (If resident is due for discharge in the near future) the resident's/representative's involvement in discharge planning.	**Notes:**

Ending Hospital Readmissions: A Blueprint for SNFs

Staff Interviews	
Interview staff on various shifts to determine: ❑ How much assistance is needed to complete ADL tasks, including transfer and ambulation. ❑ Whether the resident receives therapy or restorative services, and what is the schedule. ❑ Whether the resident is using any supportive and/or assistive devices. ❑ What restorative interventions staff are following, according to the care plan. ❑ Whether the resident displays any resistance to care, resistance to using any assistive devices, or refusal to attend therapy, and how staff respond. ❑ Whether they are aware of a plan to discharge the resident to a lesser level of care or to home in the near future (if there is such a plan).	**Notes:**

Assessment	

❑ Review the MDS, physician orders, therapy notes, consultations, and other progress notes that may have information regarding the assessment of rehabilitative and discharge needs.
❑ Based on observation of the resident, interviews with staff, and interviews with the resident/responsible party (if possible), determine whether the assessment information accurately and comprehensively reflects that status of the resident.
❑ Determine whether the assessment performs the following, as appropriate:
  • Identifies causal, contributing, and risk factors for decline or lack of improvement such as an unstable condition or an acute health problem, fracture, stroke, pain, neurological deficits, change in cognition, change in medications that may affect functional performance, and/or visual/hearing problems.
  • Identifies problems and strengths related to functional and communication skills (such as gross and fine motor coordination, sensory awareness, auditory comprehension, speech production and the use of expressive language, swallow reflex function, visual-spatial awareness, body integration, and muscle strength including balance).
  • Identifies the amount and type of assistance needed to perform rehabilitative and restorative tasks.
  • Discusses the need for, proper fit, and use of assistive devices to enable the resident to reach or maintain his or her highest level of physical function.
	Notes:

Assessment	
• Identifies history of previous refusal, resistance, or reluctance of the resident to the use of assistive devices and/or performance of exercises. • Includes an evaluation of overall medical, health, and psychosocial status to determine appropriate expectations for rehabilitation and discharge potential. • Includes a review of living arrangements prior to nursing home admission, potential for discharge, discharge needs (such as setting up home services, needed changes to the home), and possible postdischarge alternatives.	**Notes:**
1. Did the facility assess adequately to identify rehabilitative needs and potential for community discharge? ❑ Yes ❑ No F272	
*The comprehensive assessment is not required to be completed until 14 days after admission. For newly admitted residents, before the 14-day assessment is complete, the lack of sufficient assessment and care planning to meet the resident's needs should be addressed under **F281** (see the Care and Services Meet Professional Standards section).* *NOTE: The facility may have completed a five-day assessment for the Medicare beneficiary. Use the five-day assessment as the comprehensive review only if it was completed with the CAAs.*	

Care Planning	
If the care plan refers to a specific facility treatment protocol that contains details of the treatment regimen, the care plan should refer to that protocol and should clarify any deviations from or revisions to the protocol for this resident. The treatment protocol must be available to care givers, and staff should be familiar with the protocol requirements. ❑ Review the care plan to determine whether the plan is based upon the goals, needs, and strengths specific to the resident and reflects the comprehensive assessment. Determine whether the plan performs the following, as applicable: • Uses assessment information in the development of the care plan and addresses relevant risk, contributing, and causal factors. • Identifies staff/departments responsible for services (i.e., therapy, restorative, or nursing staff); interventions to be provided by staff other than therapists (e.g., nursing or restorative staff) reflective of therapy goals and interventions. • Uses interventions designed to increase resident performance and decrease the amount of staff assistance needed to perform a task. • Includes interventions that reflect the resident's medical/health condition. • (If rehabilitative therapy was discontinued), a maintenance program (provided by nursing or restorative services staff) was initiated to maintain functional and physical status, according to resident's medical/health condition. • Identifies supportive and assistive devices/equipment that is needed to meet physical and ADL needs.	**Notes:**

Ending Hospital Readmissions: A Blueprint for SNFs

Care Planning	
• Reflects (for the resident who refused or is resistant to services) efforts to find alternative means to address the needs identified in the assessment process. • Reflects resident preferences and opinions. • Includes (for a resident who is getting ready for discharge) interventions that specifically address discharge planning such as predischarge self-care and health education, review of community options, assisting with arrangements for home or community visits, and arranging for postdischarge services. ❏ If care plan concerns are noted, Interview staff responsible for care planning as to the rationale for the current plan of care.	**Notes:**
2. Did the facility develop a care plan to rehabilitative needs and other factors affecting potential for community discharge? ❏ Yes ❏ No **F279**	
*The comprehensive care plan does not need to be completed until seven days after the comprehensive assessment (the assessment completed with the CAAs). Lack of sufficient care planning to meet the needs of a newly admitted resident should be addressed under **F281** (see the Care and Services Meet Professional Standards section).* *Additionally, lack of physician orders for immediate care (until staff can conduct a comprehensive assessment and develop an interdisciplinary care plan) should be addressed under **F271**.*	

Care and Services Meet Professional Standards	
Interviews With Healthcare Practitioners and Professionals:	**Notes:**
If the interventions defined or care provided appear to not be consistent with recognized standards of practice, interview one or more healthcare practitioners and professionals (e.g., therapist, physician, charge nurse, director of nursing, social worker) who, by virtue of training and knowledge of the resident, should be able to provide information about the causes, treatment, and evaluation of the resident's condition or problem. If the attending physician is unavailable, interview the medical director, as appropriate. Depending on the issue, ask about: ❑ The causal and/or contributing factors to the problems related to functional and communication skills. ❑ How the resident's overall medical, health, and psychosocial status has affected the progress of rehabilitation, ADL improvement, and readiness for discharge. ❑ What specific services were received during therapy sessions (e.g., services to increase activity tolerance, decrease amount of staff assistance needed, improve strength and balance, improve speech, instruction on use of assistive devices). ❑ What contributed to a lack of expected improvement in functioning. ❑ The nature of the discharge plan including time frames, plans to obtain community services, family instruction in assisting the resident when at home, etc. ❑ What preparations the facility made for the resident's expected postdischarge needs (such as contacts with community service providers, evaluation of the prospective living setting to determine what changes were needed to support the resident's discharge, etc.).	
3. Did the facility implement practices that meet professional standards of quality? ❑ Yes ❑ No **F281**	
NOTE: If the care plan addressed the risks and identified needs of the resident, but the care plan was not implemented as written, consider F282 for failure to implement the care plan.	

Ending Hospital Readmissions: A Blueprint for SNFs

Care Plan Revision	
Determine whether the resident's condition and effectiveness of the care plan interventions have been monitored and care plan revisions (and discharge plan revisions, as appropriate) were made based upon the following: ❑ The outcome and/or effects of goals and interventions. ❑ A decline or lack of improvement in functioning. ❑ Intervening medical events (such as acute illness or change in health status). ❑ The resident's lack of compliance with the treatment regimen. ❑ Alternatives and/or treatment revision for refusal, resistance, or reluctance of the resident to the use of assistive devices and/or performance of exercises. ❑ Changes in the appropriateness of the discharge setting and services such as changes in availability of primary care giver, long waiting list for needed postdischarge health services.	**Notes:**
4. Did the facility revise the care plan as needed? ❑ Yes ❑ No F280	

Provision of Care and Services	
Criteria for Compliance: ❑ **F250, Social Services**—The facility is in compliance with F250 if the facility has provided adequate discharge planning based on the resident's strengths and needs, potential, and living alternatives. ❑ **F311, Activities of Daily Living**—The facility is in compliance with F311 for the provision of restorative services by nursing staff if they have given the resident the appropriate treatment and services to improve functional abilities. ❑ **F406, Specialized Rehabilitative Services**—The facility is in compliance with F406 if professional therapy staff and qualified therapy assistants have provided adequate rehabilitative services based on the resident's assessed needs and strengths according to the care plan. 5. **Based on observation, interviews, and record review did the facility ensure that (a) the resident received necessary rehabilitative services and, (b) based on discharge potential, discharge planning was provided? ❑ Yes ❑ No F280**	**Notes:**

Concerns With Structure, Process, and/or Outcome Requirements Related to Process of Care	
During the investigation, the surveyor may have identified concerns with related outcome, process, and/or structure requirements. The surveyor is cautioned to investigate these related requirements before determining whether noncompliance may be present. Some examples of requirements that should be considered include, but are not limited to, the following: ❑ **F157, Notification of Changes**—Determine whether staff notified the physician of significant changes in the resident's condition or refusal or lack of progress in the treatment plan. ❑ **F164, Privacy and Confidentiality**—Determine whether staff provide visual privacy during treatments that expose the body. ❑ **F241, Dignity**—Determine whether staff provide treatments and assistance in a manner that preserves the resident's dignity. ❑ **F242, Self-determination and Participation**—Determine whether the facility has provided the resident with choices about aspects of his or her life in the facility that are significant to the resident. ❑ **F246, Accommodation of Needs**—Determine whether the facility has adapted the resident's physical environment (room, bathroom, furniture, temperature, lighting, sound levels) to accommodate the resident's individual needs. ❑ **F309, Quality of Care**—Determine whether the resident is receiving adequate pain management. ❑ **F318, Range of Motion**—Determine whether the resident admitted with ROM limitations experienced a further decline or lack of improvement in range of motion. ❑ **F353, Sufficient Staff**—Determine whether the facility had qualified staff in sufficient numbers to provide necessary care and services, based upon the comprehensive assessment and care plan.	**Notes:**

Concerns With Structure, Process, and/or Outcome Requirements Related to Process of Care	
❏ **F385, Physician Supervision**—Determine whether the physician has assessed, evaluated, ordered, and revised orders as appropriate. ❏ **F498, Proficiency of Nurse Aides**—Determine whether nurse aides demonstrate competency in the provision of restorative nursing. ❏ **F501, Medical Director**—Determine whether the medical director: • Assisted the facility in the development and implementation of policies and procedures for rehabilitative and restorative services based on current standards of practice and policies on discharge planning. • Interacted with the physician supervising the care of the resident if requested by the facility to intervene on behalf of the resident. *If the surveyor determines that the facility is not in compliance with any of these related requirements, the appropriate Ftag should be surveyor initiated.*	Notes:

Transition Coordinator Job Description

General statement of duties

The transition coordinator completes screenings for long-term care facility applicants and makes recommendations for facility admission. When transitions are appropriate, he or she assesses residents and makes referrals to facilitate transfer to community services or alternate living arrangements based on the resident's needs. He or she is also responsible for implementing transition activities to identify long-term care facility residents who wish to return to the community and working with residents, families, long-term care facility staff, and other organizations as needed to facilitate discharge and coordinate services. This is a full-time position that may include evenings and some weekends.

Supervised by: Director of Nursing

Examples of duties:

- Identify residents who have requested, may be appropriate for, or wish to consider returning to the community through personal interviews, review of admission lists, conversion requests, referrals, and regular visits.

- Develop relationships with long-term care facility staff to encourage identification and information on residents interested in returning to the community and provide ongoing education about local and community resources.

- Performs comprehensive needs assessments, including mental, physical, functional, and environmental to determine appropriate referrals. Assesses a person's needs, determines eligibility, and takes appropriate action to initiate care or services.

- Performs assessments on individuals to determine potential for discharge. Identifies potential barriers to discharge and develops a plan to address them.

- Counsels with people entering and leaving the long-term care facility, identifies and refers to the appropriate services and funding sources.

- Upon discharge, monitors the resident's service plan in the community for 30 to 180 days as needed to ensure resources and services are sufficient to meet the former resident's needs.

- Coordinates referrals.

- Provides site visits to select persons in hospitals, rehab facilities, other long-term care facilities, potential or former residents, or families in private residences.

- Completes all paperwork and statistical reporting as required.

Qualifications:

- Licensed nurse with a minimum of three years of clinical experience. Preference will be given to a registered nurse. Long-term care facility and community nursing experience preferred.

Knowledge, skills, and abilities required

- Ability to assess a resident's specific needs and plan solutions; to understand and relate to behavior of individuals; to support the objectives and philosophy of the facility and meets the requirements of good case management.

- Develops preliminary care planning, conducts research, and provides limited follow-up.

- Interprets and transcribes medical records.

- Works as a team member.

- Follows designated instructions.

- Communicates well orally and in writing.

- Conveys difficult decisions to a resident or family in a tactful and diplomatic manner.

- Uses good interviewing, organizing, and assessment skills.

- Possesses strong knowledge of the geographical area.

- Well-versed in approved nursing techniques to observe, assess, plan, and implement a plan of care and evaluate each resident.

- Has strong assessment skills and the ability to identify the full scope of a person's needs and ability to live independently.

- Interprets information and certifies eligibility for programs and services being authorized on the post-discharge plan of care.

- Well-versed in the operation of office equipment, including but not limited to, telephone, facsimile, copy machines, printers, and computer equipment.

- Demonstrated leadership ability, strong organizational and interpersonal skills, and working knowledge of community resources and reimbursement systems for health and social services.

- Demonstrated ability to work effectively with teams of professionals representing multiple disciplines, including physicians, RNs, licensed therapists, residents, and families.

- Demonstrated ability to interact professionally and coordinate services with personnel from other facilities, agencies, and professionals in the community.

- Excellent communication skills, including the ability to educate professionals in the long-term care facility about the supports available to elders in the community.

- Performs resident assessment with PAS/PASRR programs, as appropriate.

- Refers individuals to services available through community agencies and organizations to identify options and meet the transition goals and objectives.

- Demonstrates ability to provide effective discharge teaching appropriate to culture and literacy level of residents and families.

- Visits all new admissions to begin discharge planning.

- Reports on dispositions and discharges.

- Attends staff meetings and training sessions; consults with team supervisor.

- Completes required documentation and reports in a concise manner; works closely and coordinates with other facility staff members.

- Well-versed in the various funding streams, as well as resources and programs available in the community that are beneficial to residents.

- Completes work in a quality and timely manner in accordance with program standards and guidelines, facility policies, and procedures.

- Strong work ethic.

- Ability to work independently.

- Ability to multitask effectively.

- Computer experience required.

Working relationships

- Ability to establish and maintain effective working relationships with representatives of other social agencies, institution officials, healthcare professionals, the public, and residents.

- Works with residents and families to interview and determine needs, make judgments, and convey the results of the assessment, explaining how and why a determination was made.

- Works with long-term care facility administration or staff to notify them of the approval or disapproval of admission application.

- Works with long-term care facility discharge planner, social worker, social service designee, resident, family, physicians, nursing personnel, and community health providers and agencies/organizations to develop an individualized, safe, and effective transition plan that meets the needs of each individual.

- Works with hospital discharge planners and case managers.

- Works with other community agencies to provide services to residents.

- Works with physicians to determine safe return of resident to the community or to determine safety in remaining the community.

- Exercises good judgment in evaluating situations and in making decisions.

- Writes case histories and related reports.

- Communicates effectively, summarizes data, prepares reports, and makes recommendations based on findings that contribute to solving problems and achieving work objectives.

Conditions of employment

- Valid driver's license, good driving record, access to a fully insured and dependable car required

- Successful candidate must submit to a pre-employment drug screening and a limited criminal history check

- Proof of educational credentials and/or licensing is required at time of employment

- This position has a six-month probationary period

- Must sign a noncompete agreement

- Conducts team meetings with appropriate staff

- Assists with/provides periodic public education sessions

- Attends monthly meetings with state agency staff

- Provides telephone, walk-in, or e-mail intake as needed

- Maintains an appearance appropriate to assigned duties and responsibilities

CHAPTER 8

Appendix

Discharge Planning and Home Safety...257

Hand-off Assessment to the Next Level of Care 267

Admission/Readmission Checklist 268

Change of Condition Documentation 272

Daily Nurses' Notes...273

Discharge Plan 274

Documentation Checklist: Process Guideline for Acute
Change of Condition..275

Fall Prevention Assessment...276

Intensive Monitoring Log 278

Medication Management Form..279

Nursing Assistant Communication Log...280

Nurse/CNA Communication Log...281

QA & A Audit...282

Systems Check for Physician Calls 284

ADL Focused Assessment..285

Warfarin Flow Sheet... 288

Discharge Planning and Home Safety

Environmental safety in the home is a broad topic because there are so many variables. Overwhelming environmental challenges that increase disability have been known to cause maladaptive behaviors and increase the risk of injury. Safety in the environment is determined by what environment the client is in! Primary goals for environmental safety involve a variety of factors, level of client independence, knowledge, and learning needs. It goes without saying that the environment should be free from obstacles and maximized to promote independence. The patient's ability must also be considered. Being independent should not be so exhausting that it increases the risk of falls. If this is the case, modified independence may be necessary (e.g., using a wheelchair for long distances instead of a cane or walker).

Evaluate the client and family/caregiver when making recommendations for home safety. Conduct a home visit prior to discharge whenever possible to ensure the home environment will meet the client's safety needs. Explore and identify the resources and support that will be needed during the discharge teaching/planning process. Consider the time available and cost when recommending home modifications. Recommend measures to promote safety and independence. Consult social workers and licensed therapists for referrals to community resources, as needed. Primary safety goals for discharge planning and teaching include the following:

- Promote safety and prevent falls.

- Facilitate independence as much as possible, but avoid overwhelming, tiring, or otherwise endangering the client.

- Ensure that needed durable medical equipment is available. Medicare Part B covers some durable medical items in the home. (The social worker and therapists should be able to assist you in obtaining suppliers who will bill Medicare or insurance, or may know of a charitable agency to fund supplies.)

- Evaluate the need for a full- or part-time home caregiver. (The social worker can assist with making referrals in this area as well.)

- Negotiate and communicate changes with the client and caregiver and gain their acceptance and cooperation.

- Ensure the caregiver's security in making environmental modifications and providing care.

- Ensure that physical and financial resources are available to accomplish the recommended task(s).

When evaluating the client and his or her circumstances, consider issues that increase the risk of falls. To some extent, these are personal issues, so the following list is not necessarily all inclusive.

Common risk factors that should be considered in discharge teaching include:

- Unfamiliar surroundings (such as when an elderly client will be discharging to an adult child's home)

- History of falls within the previous year

- Dizziness, unsteady gait, medication side effects, or other balance problems

- Cardiovascular disease

- Neurological disease

- Postural hypotension

- Slow reflexes

- Edema

- Recent surgery

- Paresis or paralysis

- Lower extremity injury, or venous, arterial, or diabetic ulcers, presence of a bandage, splint, or cast

- Use of a walker, cane, crutches or wheelchair

- Weakness

- Seizure disorder

- Impaired vision

- Hearing impairment

- Stiffness or immobility in joints caused by arthritis or an injury

- Spasticity

- Cognitive impairment

- Inability to understand or follow directions

- Impaired judgment (in addition to being caused by cognitive impairment, judgment can also be affected by denial of illness or disability, or embarrassment over limitations)

- Urgency or incontinence

- Intermittent episodes of diarrhea

Ending Hospital Readmissions: A Blueprint for SNFs

- Drugs with the potential to affect thought processes and mental clarity:

  – Laxative and diuretics

  – Polypharmacy or use of multiple medications

  – Other drugs, such as cardiac medications and antihypertensives

  – Drug–drug, food–drug, or supplement–drug interactions

  – Can the client take his or her medications correctly and as ordered

  – Inappropriate or slippery footwear, including stocking feet

  – Clothing of appropriate length; pants, nightgowns and robes are not too long so as to cause tripping

Consider developing a discharge teaching/planning checklist based on the following items for the family caregiver to evaluate the client's home environment for safety before agency discharge:

- Family caregivers (or others as appropriate) should routinely assess the living environment and provide preventive maintenance as needed.

- Means of getting help, if needed, such as a telephone or personal alarm system.

- Need for some type of emergency alert/call system. If the caregiver is in the home, a manual bell may be effective. These are available at most office supply stores.

- Telephones are conveniently placed so the client does not need to rush to answer the phone. Consider whether a cordless or cellular phone is the best option so the client can wear the phone on a lanyard or carry it on his or her person.

- Smoke detector(s) (also, a carbon monoxide detector is a good idea).

- Fire extinguisher(s) available.

- Working flashlights placed in convenient, accessible locations throughout the residence.

- Adequate, working outlets in a convenient location.

- Adequate ventilation, heating, and cooling.

- Windows have screens and locks.

- Doors have locks; the elderly client can manipulate the locks to open and close doors, if necessary.

- Peep hole or other means of looking outside without opening door.

- Adequate lighting without shadows or glare; easy access to light switches.

- Contrasting colors at potentially hazardous areas such as doorways and stairs.

- Adequate space between furniture.

- Eliminate clutter as much as possible; provide adequate space to move about.

- Floor surfaces even and nonslippery.

- Ability to safely move about on carpeting with or without adaptive devices. Tennis balls slipped over the back legs of a two-wheeled walker facilitate moving about on carpet.

- Eliminate throw rugs; tack or remove runners that roll or slip; tack rugs and glue vinyl flooring as appropriate. If the client uses a wheeled walker, the wheels tend to bunch and gather mats, throw rugs, and runners, creating a potentially hazardous situation.

Ending Hospital Readmissions: A Blueprint for SNFs

- Halls and doorways wide enough to accommodate a wheelchair or walker, if appropriate. The nuts holding the wheels to a wheeled walker tend to stick out, requiring more space to pass than would normally be expected, considering the width of the walker. The bathroom doors of some residences will not accommodate the width of a wheelchair and may need to be widened.

- Absence of steps or other environmental obstacles to wheelchair or walker use.

- Ramps, if needed for wheelchairs or walkers.

- Paint outside steps with a mixture of sand and paint to improve traction; consider nonslip strips, which are fastened securely. Reflective tape is also a good option.

- Handrail near all steps or stairs; handrails can be beneficial even if the individual must navigate one or two steps.

- Check carpeting on stairs to ensure it is firmly attached.

- Light switches at both ends of hallways and stairs.

- Light switch immediately inside inner and outer doors.

- Armchair or other chairs at proper height for ease of rising; elevate seats and armrests as necessary to reduce reliance on leg muscles alone, increasing stability.

- Remove or repair furniture in poor repair.

- Remove casters or secure wheels to prevent unexpected movement on beds, chairs, and other furnishings.

- Purchase a step stool with sturdy steps and handrails; discourage standing on chairs.

- Move frequently used objects to lower shelves or convenient areas.

- Furnishings arranged so the client does not have to twist when rising.

- Hot water temperature not too hot; set at water heater (low or medium setting).

- Safe telephone and electrical cords; these should not extend across the floor.

- Unobstructed doorways.

- Nonslip surface in bathroom, tub, or shower.

- Shower chair or stool.

- Adaptive bathing devices, if needed.

- Consider mounting a rack in the shower to hold needed bath items. If this is not possible, consider a small plastic bucket or plastic sifter like a child would use at the beach. These items will get wet, so determine how to drain them.

- Grab bars on toilet, tub, shower.

- Elevated toilet seat.

- Bathroom light switch readily accessible and close to the door.

- Faucet handles easy to operate; hot is always on left and cold on right.

- Safe, working stove.

- Stool next to stove or kitchen counter so the client can be seated for meal preparation.

- Additional stools for seating in other necessary areas, such as at the bathroom sink.

- Working refrigerator.

- Sturdy shelves within easy reach in needed locations.

Ending Hospital Readmissions: A Blueprint for SNFs

- Appropriate areas for chemical and medication storage.

- Evaluate clothing and footwear for safety; use low heeled shoes with nonslip bottoms; avoid shoes with slippery bottoms and stocking feet.

- Evaluate footwear to ensure it is appropriate for floor surfaces. (Leather or plastic soles on carpeting; non-slip soles for tile.)

- Lamp or lightswitch in close proximity to the bed so the client does not rise in the dark.

- Night light in bedroom, hallway, and bathroom.

- If nocturia is a problem, consider a bedside commode.

The following websites provide additional safety information:

National Patient Safety Foundation: *www.npsf.org*
Harvard Risk Management Foundation: *www.rmf.harvard.edu*
Planning for Independent Living: *www.lifelinesys.com/content/independent-living-assessment*
Injury Control Resource Information Network: *www.injurycontrol.com/icrin*

Other Concerns

Fear of falling is a serious concern in the elderly, who have a higher incidence of osteo-porosis and high risk of hip fracture, a contributing cause of mortality. Fear of falling can be debilitating and overwhelming to some individuals. Some clients will restrict all activity to a small area for fear of sliding on tile or using stairs. The self-imposed isola-tion can cause weakness and loss of mobility over time. Remember that falls going to or from the bathroom account for many falls in the disabled and aging. Focus on environ-mental modifications that take the urgent need for toileting into consideration.

Falls are common in the elderly and account for many emergency room visits. It is estimated that one-third to one-half of all elderly individuals are at risk of falls. Many of those who have fallen will fall again within the next six months. The onset of increased fall risk of can be gradual or sudden. A sudden increase in risk of falls usually occurs as a result of medical illness and hospitalization. Sometimes the risk of falls is gradual, such as in the insidious onset of poor perception, posture, and balance. Aging changes are often cumulative, with one problem potentiating the others. Promptly recognizing these changes and modifying the environment to prevent injury is an ongoing process.

Wandering behavior

For clients with wandering behavior, the following approaches may be effective:

- Make sure the residence is well-lighted, particularly at night.

- Tack loud jingle bells above doors.

- Install slide bolt locks at the top and/or bottom of doors. Cognitively impaired individuals seldom look up or down.

- Purchase a "baby monitor" or infant intercom system.

- Consider battery alarms that hang from the door knob and sound an alarm when the door is opened. (These are usually sold for travelers to use in hotel rooms).

- Infrared sensor alarms may be installed on the bedroom door or exit doors.

- Pressure sensitive pads that sound an alarm when the client rises from bed or chair are excellent devices to use at night.

- Pressure sensitive mats are available to place on the floor next to the bed, or the bedroom doorway. These sound an alarm if the client steps on them.

- Childproof door covers can be purchased that prevent door knobs from turning.

- Toddler monitors are available that sound an alarm if the individual wanders outside a certain distance, usually 20 to 40 feet.

- Placing dark tile on the floor approximately 2 to 3 feet in front of a doorway may be helpful. Many individuals perceive this dark area as a hole and will not cross it due to the spatial-perceptual changes caused by dementia.

- Install baby locks on cupboards where medications, chemicals, and hazardous substances are stored.

- Post signs and labels on doors, cupboards, drawers, and common rooms.

- Cover doorways with floor length curtains.

- Install one or more child safety gates a foot above the floor. Avoid using the low safety gates for individuals who may attempt to climb over them. In this case, the gates increase the risk of injury. Gates up to five feet high are available in department stores. The WalMart online catalog has a good variety. Refer to *http://tinyurl.com/2epf9xe*

- Paint exit doors the same color as surrounding walls.

- Install full length mirrors on the inside of exit doors.

- Install fences in the yard that are difficult to climb over.

- Lock outside gates.

Always consider the possibility of another type of emergency, such as fire. When modifying the residence for wandering safety, make sure you have a plan to exit the home.

Hand-off Assessment to the Next Level of Care

Yes	No	Medical Issue
		Does the resident have a primary care physician (PCP)? (If appropriate) send assessment information to PCP – Date
		Does the resident have a specialty physician (e.g., cardiologist)? (If appropriate) send assessment information – Date
		Does the resident have a psychiatrist or other mental health provider? (If appropriate) send assessment information – Date
		Does the resident have an outpatient case manager who should be notified? Send assessment information – Date
		Ensure all transition services and care (medications, equipment, home care, SNF, hospice) are coordinated and documented – Date verified
		Ensure resident and caregiver understand all information and have a copy of the care plan with them – Date verified

Client name: _____

Ending Hospital Readmissions: A Blueprint for SNFs

Admission/Readmission Checklist

Resident Name: _____   Date: _____

Admission/Readmission Checklist

Item	Initials	Date	Comments
Resident ID Band			
HIPAA Consents signed for name, photos, etc.			*Note restrictions:*
Bed (and/or door frame) Labeled per policy			
Showed resident how to use call signal			
Admission Nursing History Complete			
Complete skin check			
Immunization history completed; consents signed			
Personal Inventory			
Belongings Labeled			
Dentures marked			
Jewelry described; release to keep at bedside signed or sent home/locked in safe			*Note description of jewelry if release signed. If not, note disposition.*
History & Physical			
Discharge Summary			
Transfer Form			
Advance Directive			
Consent-CPR/DNR			
Consent-Rails and Restraints			
Consent-Smoking			
Fall Risk Assessment			
Skin Risk Assessment			
Other Assessment (Specify)			
Other Assessment (Specify)			
Care Plan Initiated			
Diet ordered			
Admission Lab ordered			

Admission/Readmission Checklist (cont.)

Give first step Mantoux; schedule reading			
Chest x-ray ordered			
Therapy consults requested, if indicated			
Admission nursing note			Document date and time of admission, from where, transportation, room number, overall condition, mental status, summary of primary diagnosis, skin condition, complete vital signs, allergies, notifications.
Schedule for nursing notes/vitals q shift x 72h			
Height/weight obtained			
Schedule appointments			
Add to bath schedule			
Initiate intake and output monitoring, if indicated			
Admission orders			
Diagnosis			Medications; include diagnosis for each
PRN			Define PRN orders (for what, when)
Diet			Diet
Activities			Activities per plan of care
Rehab potential			Rehab potential/prognosis
Therapy			Therapy evaluations, if indicated; treat per plan of care
Mantoux			Two-step Mantoux testing or chest X-Ray
Pass			May go on therapeutic pass with medications PRN, or as indicated
POD prn			Podiatrist, optometrist, dentist PRN
Foley			Foley catheter-size and orders to change; obtain order to remove, if indicated
Tube feeding			Tube feeding type, size; orders to change for plugging or accidental dislodgment, if indicated
			• Tube feeding solution, type of administration, time, amount, number of calories per day
			• Obtain orders for free water on all tube feeders, including 30 to 50 ml before and after each medication
			• Obtain orders for tube placement checks, residual checks
			• Measure and document length of tube
			• List HOB elevation, other special care on care plan
			• Obtain a physician's order if the continuous tube feeding must be suspended for any reason; for example, a daily shower. (Or obtain an order to run continuous feeding 23 hours a day to allow for ADL care)

Ending Hospital Readmissions: A Blueprint for SNFs

Admission/Readmission Checklist (cont.)

Weight and Vitals			Specify frequency of weight and vital signs on physician order sheet
Communicable disease			Note resident is free from communicable disease
Informed of condition			Note that resident or legal representative have been apprised of resident's condition
Fingerstick blood sugar			If resident is diabetic, note frequency for blood sugar testing. Specify physician notification for blood sugar above 300 and below 70, or according to policy.
Medication Monitoring			If resident is on Coumadin (warfarin), note frequency for INR and protime testing
			• Inquire about specific laboratory testing related to medications (e.g., digoxin, anti-seizure medications, lithium, etc.)
Ancillary orders			Obtain routine orders per facility policy (laxative, medication for pain/fever, skin tear treatment, etc.)
Treatment orders			Obtain specific treatment orders (area, frequency, stop order or until healed)
Oxygen			If resident is using oxygen, note liter flow, method, and frequency
Restraints, including siderails			Type, time, reason, release.
Physician contacted; Orders verified			
Allergies documented on MAR, chart cover, and as indicated			
ADL Sheet started			
Pharmaceuticals Ordered			
MAR started			
Treatment Record started			
Other, according to facility policy:			

Admission/Readmission Checklist (cont.)

Item	Date Obtained	Initials	Comments
History & Physical			
CBC			
Hemoglobin			
Hematocrit			
Chemistry			
Glucose			
BUN			
Creatinine			
Urinalysis			
Stool for Occult Blood			
PPD Step 1			
PPD Step 2			
Chest x-ray			
Vision exam			
Hearing exam			
Dental exam			
Immunizations - Pneumovax (5 years)			
Immunizations - Influenza			
Immunizations - DT (10 years)			
Other Assessment (Specify)			
Other Assessment (Specify)			

Ending Hospital Readmissions: A Blueprint for SNFs

Change of Condition Documentation

Instructions: Document in the nurses' notes on the conditions listed below for a minimum of 72 hours or until complete resolution. Complete and document at least one focused, systemic assessment every shift, or more often.

	Condition	Date/Time of Onset
❑	New Admission	
❑	Antibiotics (Assess and document reason(s) for treatment)	
❑	Vital signs T P R B/P Pulse Oximeter	
❑	Cough, congestion, URI	
❑	Nausea, vomiting	
❑	Diarrhea, loose stools	
❑	Abdominal pain	
❑	Change in diet, appetite, eating habits	
❑	Pressure ulcer	
❑	Skin tear, laceration, abrasion	
❑	Rash, redness, warmth or other skin eruption	
❑	Edema	
❑	Urinary frequency, pain, burning, etc. or diagnosed UTI	
❑	Abnormal behavior (new onset)	
❑	Change in mental status	
❑	Change in level of consciousness	

❑	Incident, injury, or fall
	    ❑ Fall
	    ❑ Skin tear
	    ❑ Bruise
	    ❑ Other injury (specify):	

❑	Wandered out (eloped)	
❑	Other, specify:	
❑	Other, specify:	
❑	Other, specify:	
❑	Other, specify:	

_____   _____   _____
       Resident Name   **Room No.**   **Physician**

_____   _____
    Signature of Nurse Initiating Form   **Date**

Daily Nurses' Notes

Resident: _____ Date: _____

DAILY NURSES' NOTES

Skin Check	N	D	E
Warm to touch?			
Cool to touch? *			
Dry?			
Clammy? *			
Diaphoretic? *			
Color normal			
Pale? *			
Dusky? *			
Cyanotic? *			
Turgor (G, F*, P*)			
Mucous Membranes			

Safety Check	N	D	E
Bed in low position?			
Side rails up?			
Call signal in reach			
Restrained correctly, if ordered			

Diabetic Record			
	Time	FSBS	Ketone/Acetone
N			
D			
E			

	Fluid Intake	Fluid Ouput
N		
D		
E		

Signatures	
N	
D	
E	

Radial Pulses	N	D	N
Strong			
Weak *			
Absent *			
= Bilat			
> on Right *			
> on Left *			

Pedal Pulses	N	D	E
Strong			
Weak *			
Absent *			
= Bilat			
> on Right *			
> on Left *			

* **NOTE:** All abnormal conditions (**) must be described in Nurses' Notes. A narrative note is required for all ** conditions.

Lungs	N	D	E
Clear R			
Clear L			
Coarse **			
Wheezes **			
Rales (Crackles) **			

Edema	N	D	E
No edema present			
Non-pitting **			
Pitting **			

*NOTE: Any edema must be documented in Nurses' Notes, describing location and quantifying degree 1˚, 2˚, 3˚, or 4˚.

Care/Activity	N	D	E
Bathed?			
Oral hygiene?			
Peri Care?			
Skin Care?			
Tube Care? (Use flow sheet)			
Turned as ordered?			
BSC or BRP ?			
Up in chair or W/C?			
Ambulated (self)?			
Ambulated with assist			

Abdomen	N	D	E
Soft			
Flat			
Distended *			
Taut *			

Abdominal Sounds	N	D	E
Active			
Hyper *			
Hypo *			
Absent *			

Sensorium/ Oriented to:	N	D	E
Time			
Place			
Person			

*NOTE: Document sensorium/mental status only if it varies from resident's normal.

* Note: All abnormal findings on this record require a narrative note in the Nurses' Notes.

Ending Hospital Readmissions: A Blueprint for SNFs

Discharge Plan

§483.15(g)(1) The facility must provide medically-related social services to attain or maintain the highest practicable physical, mental, and psychosocial well-being of each resident. Discharge planning services include helping to place a resident on a waiting list for community congregate living, arranging intake for home care services for residents returning home, and assisting with transfer arrangements to other facilities.

Dear Doctor: Please complete the (tentative) discharge plan on your resident,
_____ _____within seven days and return it to us by: _____.
Thank you!

Discharge Plan	Yes	No
Resident will be discharging to:		
a. Own home or home of a relative		
b. Intermediate care facility		
c. Sheltered or residential care facility		
d. Other, specify:		
e. Prolonged or permanent placement in this facility anticipated		
If resident is discharging to home, he or she will need:		
Personal care		
Nursing services		
Housekeeping assistance		
Adaptive equipment or medical supplies		
Assistance with psychosocial or emotional adjustment		
Dietitian		
Physical Therapy		
Occupational Therapy		
Speech Therapy		
Respiratory Therapy		
Community resources or services (specify):		
Financial assistance		
Other, specify:		
Other, specify:		
None of the above		
I will be making discharge plans and providing related services to this patient.		
I would appreciate facility staff assistance with discharge planning.		
Physician Signature	Date:	

Ending Hospital Readmissions: A Blueprint for SNFs

Documentation Checklist: Process Guideline
for Acute Change of Condition

ACUTE CHANGE OF CONDITION: Assessment/Problem Recognition			
May relate to F-tag: 272 (Assessment), 309 (Quality of Care)	Yes	No	NA
1. Did the facility identify significant risks for an ACOC?			
2. Did the facility describe and document symptoms and/or conditions changes?			
3. Did the facility clarify the nature of the problem?			

ACUTE CHANGE OF CONDITION: Diagnosis/Cause Identification			
May relate to F-tag: 272 (Assessment, 385 (Physician services), 386 (Physician review of total plan of care)	Yes	No	NA
4. Did the facility staff and practitioner seek causes of the symptoms or condition change, or can they justify sending the individual out of the facility to evaluate possible causes?			
5. If a plausible cause was not found readily in someone with an ACOC, were delirium, fluid and electrolyte imbalance, infection, and medication-related effects considered?			

ACUTE CHANGE OF CONDITION: Treatment/Problem Management			
May relate to F-tag: 279/280 (Comprehensive Care Plans), 309 (Quality of Care), 386 (Physician review of total plan of care)	Yes	No	NA
6. Did the facility address the ACOC or identify why it was not appropriate to do so, and review as part of its QA process why it was necessary to send an individual elsewhere to address an ACOC?			
7. Was appropriate supportive and cause-specific treatment given OR was there an explanation why it was not feasible or not provided?			

ACUTE CHANGE OF CONDITION: Monitoring			
May relate to F-tag: 272 (Assessment), 309 (Quality of Care)	Yes	No	NA
8. Were the individual's ACOC and related causes monitored and treatment adjusted accordingly?			
9. Does the facility monitor its unplanned hospital transfers as part of its QA program and seek to improve on related processes?			

Signature of Person(s) completing the form:

_____   _____

Signature   Date

_____   _____

Signature   Date

Ending Hospital Readmissions: A Blueprint for SNFs

Fall Prevention Assessment

Resident Name: _____ Room: _____ Assessment Date: _____

Fall Prevention Assessment

Instructions: Complete this form on admission and each time an MDS is done.

Part I.
❐ Over age 75
❐ Agitation
❐ Confusion, memory impairment, judgment impairment, delirium, dementia
❐ Unwilling or unable to follow instructions
❐ Dizziness or vertigo
❐ Previous history of falls
❐ Incontinence
❐ Frequently needs to use toilet
❐ Hypovolemia or orthostasis
❐ New to facility/new admission within the past 30 days
❐*Other (according to QA & A Committee guidelines and protocols):* _____
_____
❐ _____

If any of the boxes are checked in Part I, the resident is at risk for falls. Initiate and implement a fall prevention plan of care.

Part II.
❐ Takes any of the following: Anticonvulsants, antidepressants, antihypertensives, sedatives, hypnotic, tranquilizers, diuretics, laxatives, eye drops
❐ Muscle weakness or paralysis
❐ Depression
❐ Restricted by equipment or tubing (Foley, IV, oxygen, feeding tube, etc.)
❐ Requires assistance with ambulation OR has unsteady gait OR uses cane or walker
❐ History or seizures OR any past history of neurological diagnoses (MS, polio, Parkinson's, etc.)
❐ Poor or uncorrected vision
❐ Poor or uncorrected hearing
❐ Peripheral vascular disease, peripheral neuropathy, or impaired sensation
❐ Inability to communicate or make needs known
❐ *Other (according to QA & A Committee guidelines and protocols):*
❐ _____
❐ _____

If two or more of the boxes are checked in Part II, the resident is at risk for falls. Initiate and implement a fall prevention plan of care.

❐ Resident is at risk for falls   ❐ Resident is not at risk for falls at this time

_____   _____

Assessed by (Nurse)_____ Date_____Time_____

Fall Prevention Assessment (cont.)

Fall Prevention Plan of Care

Instructions: Check all precautions initiated and care planned for this resident.

Bed/Call Signal
❏ Bed in low position with wheels locked
❏ Call signal within reach
❏ Side rails up x _____
❏ Bed exit alarm applied
❏ Low bed
❏ Matt on floor next to bed
❏ Adaptive devices (body pillow, bolsters, etc.) Specify device(s): _____

Communication
❏ Paper and pen
❏ Communication board
❏ Manual call bell
❏ Other, specify: _____

Request Consultations:
❏ Physical Therapy
❏ Occupational Therapy
❏ Social Service or Mental Health
❏ Evaluate footwear for proper fit, appropriateness of sole to floor surface, etc.
❏ Other, specify: _____

Education:
❏ Resident and family teaching, specify: _____
❏ Staff teaching, specify: _____
❏ Activity restrictions
❏ Other, specify: _____

Vision and hearing:
❏ Glasses clean and on
❏ Hearing aid on and working

Immediate Environment:
❏ Pathway to bathroom free of obstacles
❏ Minimum furniture and equipment in room
❏ Room kept tidy
❏ Bathroom light on at night
❏ Door/blinds open at all times
❏ Room near nurses' station

Medical Condition:
❏ Routine blood pressure and pulse checks q _____
❏ Orthostatic blood pressure checks q _____

Mobility:
❏ Bedside commode
❏ Take to bathroom or toilet according to individual schedule
❏ Gait belt/transfer belt
❏ Mechanical lift
❏ Number of staff to transfer _____
❏ Cane, walker, wheelchair for ambulation. Specify which: _____

❏ Fall prevention armband (specify color): _____
❏ Visual check q _____
❏ Other, specify: _____

Ending Hospital Readmissions: A Blueprint for SNFs

Intensive Monitoring Log

Resident Name: _____   Date: _____

Intensive Monitoring Log

Purpose/reason intensive monitoring is necessary:_____

_____

Time	Location	Activity/Observation	Initials	Time	Location	Activity/Observation	Initials
12 AM				12 AM			
1 AM				1 AM			
2 AM				2 AM			
3 AM				3 AM			
4 AM				4 AM			
5 AM				5 AM			
6 AM				6 AM			
7 AM				7 AM			
8 AM				8 AM			
9 AM				9 AM			
10 AM				10 AM			
11 AM				11 AM			
12 PM				12 PM			
1 PM				1 PM			
2 PM				2 PM			
3 PM				3 PM			
4 PM				4 PM			
5 PM				5 PM			
6 PM				6 PM			
7 PM				7 PM			
8 PM				8 PM			
9 PM				9 PM			
10 PM				10 PM			
11 PM				11 PM			

Medication Management Form

Name: _____

Date List Prepared or Updated: _____

Pharmacy Name and Address: _____

Pharmacy Phone: _____

Medication name (brand or generic)	Dosage	When to take (number of times per day, time, special instructions)	Reason (why taking it)	Start date	Stop date	Monitoring needed (check pulse, weekly lab test, etc.)	Prescribed by	Side effects, danger signs, things to watch for

Over-the-Counter (OTC) Drugs Used:
- Allergy relief, antihistamines
- Antacids
- Baby aspirin
- Cold/Cough
- Diet
- Herbs
- Laxatives/Softeners
- Pain Medications
- Sleep Aids
- Vitamins/Minerals

Other (List):
_____
_____
_____
_____
_____

Ending Hospital Readmissions: A Blueprint for SNFs

Nursing Assistant Communication Log

NA Name: Resident Name: Date:

Time	T	P	R	B/P	Mark Skin Problems on Diagram

Height	Weight				

Elimination					
Urination	Continent	Incontinent	How Many?	Abnormalities	
BM-Large	BM-Medium	BM-Small	No BM	Abnormalities	

General Information	
Bath	
Nails done	
Oral Care	
Skin Condition-Be specific! (hydrated, abnormalities, etc.)	
Assistance with ambulation	
Protective safety device (if any) applied and released	

Indicate Ulcer Sites:

Anterior   Posterior
(Attach a color photo of the pressure ulcer(s) [Optional])

Fluid Consumption				
Good	Fair	Poor	Intake, if ordered	Output, if ordered

Meal Consumption (Circle One)					
Breakfast	Good	Fair	Poor	Substitute?	Refused/Comment
Lunch	Good	Fair	Poor	Substitute?	Refused/Comment
AM Snack	Good	Fair	Poor	Refused	Comment
PM Snack	Good	Fair	Poor	Refused	Comment

Attitude/Mental Condition (Circle One)				Comments, Concerns, Issues to Report to Nurse
Sad	Happy	Sleepy	Other (Specify)	
Comment:				

Activities, if any

Nurse/CNA Communication Log

CNA: Resident Name: Date:

6-2						2-10					
Vital Signs:						Vital Signs:					
Time	T	P	R	B/P	02	RSI	Time	T	P	R	B/P	02	RSI

BM's		BM's	

General Info	General Info

OOB:

PT Programs:
ROM
Ambulate
AFO's On
Body Jacket On
OT Programs:
Oral Stim
Hand Splints On
Feeding Issues

Meal Consumption:
Good   Fair   Poor
Good   Fair   Poor

Fluid Consumption:
Good   Fair   Poor
Good   Fair   Poor

Menses:
Heavy   Moderate   Light   Scant

HS:

OOB:

PT Programs:
ROM
Ambulate
AFO's On
Body Jacket On
OT Programs:
Oral Stim
Hand Splints On
Feeding Issues:

Meal Consumption:
Good   Fair   Poor
Good   Fair   Poor

Fluid Consumption:
Good   Fair   Poor
Good   Fair   Poor

Menses:
Heavy   Moderate   Light   Scant

HS:

Other Info (Phone calls, behaviors)	Other Info (Phone calls, behaviors)

Ending Hospital Readmissions: A Blueprint for SNFs

QA & A Audit

Subject of audit: _____

OBRA REQUIREMENT NUMBER (§_____)

TAG NUMBER(S): F_____, F_____, F_____,
F_____, F_____, F_____, F_____, F_____, F_____,

QUALITY INDICATORS:

1. Administrative rules and regulations

2. Provision of staff and services to residents by those within and outside the facility

DATE:

DATE COMPLETED:

RESIDENT/SAMPLE SIZE:

SOURCES OF INFORMATION:

1. Investigation of compliance with laws and professional standards
2. Investigation of qualifications and services furnished by outside providers
3. Medical record review
4. Systems review
5. Direct observation
6. Other
   _____

QUALITY ACTION TEAM MEMBERS:

1. Administrator
2. Director of Nursing
3. Infection Control Nurse
4. Nurse Manager and/or Quality Improvement Coordinator
5. Representative from outside provider
6. Other:
   _____

   _____

Response Codes	Yes=X	No=0		Not Applicable =									
Criteria						Resident Number							
		1	2	3	4	5	6	7	8	9	10
I.											
II.											
III.											
IV.											
V.											
VI.											
VII.											
VIII.											
IX.											
X.											
XI.											
XII.											
XIII.											
XIV.											

Ending Hospital Readmissions: A Blueprint for SNFs

QA & A Audit (cont.)

Response Codes	Yes=X	No=0	Not Applicable =									
Criteria						Resident Number						
	1	2	3	4	5	6	7	8	9	10
XV.										
XVI.										
XVII.										
XVIII.										
XIX.										
XX.										
XXI.										
XXII.										
XXIII.										
XXIV.										
XXV.										
XXVI.										
XXVII.										
XXVIII.										
XXIX.										

SUMMARY OF RESULTS OF AUDIT:

Problems/deficiencies identified:_____

_____

Reasons for problems:_____

_____

Actions planned or taken:_____

_____

Correction of problems or
deficiencies:_____

_____

Alternatives or revisions of
procedure:_____

_____

Ending Hospital Readmissions: A Blueprint for SNFs

Systems Check for Physician Calls

Instructions: Prior to placing a call to the physician change, you must perform a systems check. Obtain the information below. File a copy of the form in the medical record.

Resident Name:		Age:	Weight:	Date:

Temp.	Pulse	Resp.	B/P	Pulse Ox	Time:

Note: Use tympanic, oral, or rectal temp. Avoid the axillary method unless other methods cannot be used.

DIAGNOSES

CURRENT MEDICATIONS

PRN Meds used past 24 hours:

Reason(s) for calling physician:

Resident has a cough: Yes   No   Productive: Yes   No   Dry: Yes   No   Moist: Yes   No

Lung Sounds

Right	Left	Edema: Yes No	Cyanosis: Yes No

Abdominal pain: Yes   No   Last BM: Check for Impaction: Yes   No

Bowel Sounds

RUQ:	LUQ:	RLQ:	LLQ:

Dietary Intake Past 24 Hours (Percentage Consumed)

AM:	NOON:	PM:

Fluid Balance, Intake Past 24 Hours

Intake:	Output:	Turgor:	Voiding:

Urine color, clarity, appearance, odor:

Mucous membranes:	Color, overall appearance:

Skin Condition

Open areas, pressure ulcers:

Mental Status

Alert: Yes   No   Confused: Yes   No   Lethargic: Yes   No   Unresponsive: Yes   No

Is mental status normal for resident?   Yes   No   Glasgow Coma Score, if head injury, CVA/TIA:

Miscellaneous/Other Observations/Relevant Information

Allergies:

Date/Time of Call: Physician: Nurse Signature:

Responsible Party/Family Notified?   Yes   No   Care Plan Updated?   Yes   No

Ending Hospital Readmissions: A Blueprint for SNFs

ADL Focused Assessment

Resident name:	Date:
Memory: __ Alert and oriented x3 __ Alert but disoriented to _____ __ Not alert __ Short term memory loss __ Long term memory loss __ No change in past 90 days __ Improved in past 90 days __ Deteriorated in past 90 days **Decision making ability:** 0 no problem I moderate impairment 2 severe impairment __ Unable to assess	**Delirium:** __Easily Distracted __Lethargy __ Altered Perception __Mental function varies __ Disorganized Speech __ Restlessness __ Delusions __ Hallucinations

Nutrition:
Diet: _____
Weight: _____   __ Weight in IBW
__ Increase past 90 days   __ Decrease past 90 days
__ Own teeth   __ Edentulous
__ Dentures   __ Upper
__ Lower   __ Partial
__ Dental implant   __ Dental problem
__ Independent   __ Total dependent
__ Adaptive device   __ Cues/set up
__ Limited assist eating   __ Extensive assist
__ Hx swallowing problems __ Corrected by diet
__ Difficulty swallowing   __ Chewing problem
__ Thickened liquids   __ Feeding tube
__ Planned weight loss   __ Supplements
Comments: _____
	Bowel and Bladder Continence:
	Total incontinence
	       __ Bowel __ Bladder __ Both
	__ Occasionally incontinent
	       __ Bowel __ Bladder __ Both
	__ Frequently incontinent
	       __ Bowel __ Bladder __ Both
	__ Scheduled toileting plan
	__ Bowel and bladder retraining
	__ Continent, independent
	__ Continent, needs assistance
	__ Catheter
	       __ External __ Indwelling __ Suprapubic
	       __ Intermittent __ Self __ Briefs/pads
	__ Ostomy
	       Type: _____
	Comments: _____

Vision: __ Adequate __ Moderately impaired __ Severely impaired __ Legally blind __ Glasses __ Contacts __ Implant __ Artificial eye __ Unable to assess, unknown Comments: _____ _____ _____	**Activities of Daily Living:** __ Independent (except showers) __ Supervision/set up __ Limited assistance __ Extensive assistance __ Total dependence __ Task segmentation __ No change in past 90 days __ Improved in past 90 days __ Deteriorated in past 90 days

Ending Hospital Readmissions: A Blueprint for SNFs

ADL Focused Assessment (cont.)

Communication and Hearing:
__ Hearing WNL
__ Minimal hearing problem
__ Moderate hearing problem
__ Severe hearing problem
__ Hearing aid _____ ear(s)
__ Unable to hear
__ Aphasia
__ Speech clear, intelligible
__ Mild to moderate speech impediment
__ Unintelligible
__ Speaks English   Other language: _____
__ Communication aid
__ Always understands communication
__ Sometimes understands communication
__ Rarely understands communication
__ Never understands communication
__ Can express needs independently
__ Minimal difficulty expressing needs
__ Moderate difficulty expressing needs
__ Severe difficulty expressing needs
__ Complete inability to express needs

Mobility, Transfers, and Ambulation:
__ Independent with all ambulation
__ Supervision needed with ambulation
__ Limited assistance needed for ambulation
__ Extensive assistance needed for ambulation
__ Unable to ambulate
__ Ambulates with assistive device
__ Propels wheelchair independently
__ Wheelchair, dependent
__ Bedfast
__ Mechanical lift
__ Independent with transfers
__ Supervision with transfers
__ Limited assist with transfers
__ Extensive assist with transfers
__ Orthotic device
__ ¼ bed mobility rail
__ ½ bed mobility rail
__ Independent bed mobility
__ Dependent bed mobility
Comments: _____
_____

Rehab Program:
__ Physical therapy
__ Occupational therapy
__ Speech therapy
__ Rehab assistant program with __ PT __ OT __ ST
__ Restorative nursing program 6 days/week or more
Describe: _____
_____
Balance: __ Sitting __ Standing
0-independent 1-unsteady; 2-partial support
3-unable to attempt without physical help
Comments: _____

Walking When Most Self Sufficient:
Farthest Distance Walked Without Sitting:

0- 50+feet   1- 51-149 ft   2- 26-50ft.
3- 10-25 ft.   4- less than 10 ft.

Time walked without sitting down during this episode:
0- 1-2min   1- 3-4 min   2- 5-10 min
3- 10-15 min   4- 16-30min   5- 31+min

__ Used ambulation aid
   Type: _____

Behavior:
__ Aggression, not easily altered
__ No change in past 90 days
__ Improved in past 90 days
__ Deteriorated in past 90 days
__ Behavior care plan in place
Comments: _____
_____
_____
_____

Contractures:
__ None
__ Present:
   __ Left arm __ Right arm __ Left leg __ Right leg
   __ Neck __ Foot __ Ankle
__ Present, other location: _____
__ Voluntary movement
__ Resists ROM
__ Splints/orthotics used for contracture management
__ Task segmentation
__ Prevention care plan in place

Psychosocial status:
__ Mood easily altered
__ Mood not easily altered
__ Psychotropic drugs
__ No change in past 90 days
__ Improved in past 90 days
__ Deteriorated in past 90 days

Edema:
__ None present
__ Present
   Location of edema: _____
_____
Comments: _____

ADL Focused Assessment (cont.)

Falls:
__ No falls past 30 days   __ 180 days
__ Fall, no injury past 30 days   __ 180 days
__ Fall with injury past 30 days __ 180 days
   Describe injuries: _____
_____
Fall prevention methods used: _____
_____
_____
__ Prevention care plan in place
Comments: _____
_____

Restraints and alternatives:
__ None
__ Restraints used:
   State type, when, why: _____
_____
__ Body alarm   __ Bed alarm   __ Chair alarm
__ No siderails used
__ Resident requests siderails up
__ Reason for rails: _____
__ Siderail up on one side
__ Bed next to wall
__ Low bed used

Skin Condition, Pressure Ulcers
__ No skin breakdown
__ Pressure ulcer:
   Location: _____
__ Stage I __ Stage II __ Stage III __ Stage IV
__ Weekly skin assessment
__ High risk for breakdown
__ Prevention care plan in place
__ Turned q2h and PRN
__ Pressure-relieving device:
   __ Bed __ Chair __ Both
   Device used: _____
__ Wound, dressing or treatment:
   Type: _____

Skin Condition, Injuries
__ Bruise(s)
   Location: _____
__ Senile purpura
   Location: _____
__ Petechiae
   Location: _____
__ Skin tear(s)
   Location: _____
Prevention methods used: _____
__ Prevention care plan in place
Other comments: _____

Pain:
__ None
__ Pain daily
__ Pain less than daily
__ Regular pain medication
   Describe pain location and intensity: _____

Medications:
__ New meds past 90 days
__ Dosage change past 90 days
   Describe: _____

Respiratory Status:
__ No problem
__ Dyspnea
__ COPD, CHF, other _____
__ Regular use of oxygen at ____ LPM
   When: _____
__ Uses nebulizer or other treatment:
   What, when: _____

Activities:
__ Room activities
__ Group activities:
   __ Active participant __ Passive participant
__ Naps during day
Comment: _____

Discharge plan:
__ No discharge potential
__ Plans to return home
__ Plans to discharge to other setting
   Where: _____
__ No change in self sufficiency past 90 days
__ Improved in self sufficiency past 90 days
__ Deteriorated in self sufficiency past 90 days
__ Active discharge plan in place

Signatures, Comments:

Ending Hospital Readmissions: A Blueprint for SNFs

Warfarin Flow Sheet

All Entries must be dated, timed and signed
Reference Value for CoagChek (0.8 – 1.4 INR)

Date	Time	PT (seconds)	INR	Warfarin Dose Ordered	Warfarin Dose Administered	RN administering Signature Double Check
						✓✓
						✓✓
						✓✓
						✓✓
						✓✓
						✓✓
						✓✓
						✓✓
						✓✓
						✓✓
						✓✓
						✓✓
						✓✓
						✓✓
						✓✓
						✓✓ ✓✓

✓✓ = double check

Ending Hospital Readmissions: A Blueprint for SNFs